Deciding Together

Deciding Together

Bioethics and Moral Consensus

Jonathan D. Moreno, Ph.D.

Professor of Pediatrics and of Medicine
Director, Division of Humanities in Medicine
SUNY Health Science Center at Brooklyn

New York   Oxford
OXFORD UNIVERSITY PRESS   1995

Oxford University Press

Oxford   New York
Athens   Auckland   Bangkok   Bombay
Calcutta   Cape Town   Dar es Salaam   Delhi
Florence   Hong Kong   Istanbul   Karachi
Kuala Lumpur   Madras   Madrid   Melbourne
Mexico City   Nairobi   Paris   Singapore
Taipei   Tokyo   Toronto

and associated companies in
Berlin   Ibadan

Copyright © 1995 by Jonathan D. Moreno

Published by Oxford University Press, Inc.,
200 Madison Avenue, New York, New York 10016

Oxford is a registered trademark of Oxford University Press

Library of Congress Cataloging-in-Publication Data
Moreno, Jonathan D.
Deciding together : bioethics and moral consensus / Jonathan D. Moreno.
p. cm.   Includes index.
ISBN 0-19-509218-X
1. Bioethics.
2. Ethics committees.
I. Title.
R724.M677   1995
174'.2—dc20   94-26756

1 3 5 7 9 8 6 4 2

Printed in the United States of America
on acid-free paper

For Jarrett Alexander Moreno

And in memory of Jacob Levy Moreno, M.D.

> "And it comes upon me strangely,
> in bidding you farewell,
> how a life is but a day,
> and expresses mainly but a single note."
>> —William James, in his last letter to his father

Acknowledgments

Many colleagues in philosophy and bioethics have participated in the development of my thinking about this subject. Andy Altman helped me formulate the initial problematic, criticized drafts of several chapters, and was wonderfully supportive and helpful throughout this project. David DeGrazia, Laurence McCullough, Stephen Wear, Ruth Macklin, John Arras, Bruce Jennings, and Jeffrey Blustein also commented on previous drafts, and I benefited from conversations with Paul Churchill and Bill Griffith. Extensive comments from several anonymous reviewers prompted me to perform radical surgery on earlier drafts.

H. Tristram Engelhardt, Jr., nursed me through revisions of my first paper on consensus in bioethics for the *Journal of Medicine and Philosophy*; were it not for Tris's encouragement, I might have dropped the project at that time. Some ideas that appear in the final document were honed in discussions at the Hastings Center, Montefiore Medical Center, and the SUNY Health Science Center at Brooklyn. I have learned much about bioethical issues from conversations with my colleagues in the Division of Humanities in Medicine, Kathleen Powderly, Connie Zuckerman, and Alice Herb. Jeffrey House of Oxford University Press stuck with me through the several extensive revisions and at each stage recruited a number of superb reviewers.

Much of the research for this book was conducted at the National Reference Center for Bioethics Literature of the National Library of Medicine. I am grateful to several members of their superb staff for their assistance in tracking down various materials.

My family's contribution, and especially that of my wife, cannot be adequately acknowledged. In the long course of writing this book my children acquired the uncanny discipline not to roll, crawl, toddle, or run (depending on the prevailing developmental stage) into my study while I was working, or at least not to do so too often. Leslye insisted on finding time for me to write, even (and perhaps especially) when I was decidedly disinclined to do so. While pursuing her own demanding career, she has been able to provide the love and support that sustain all of us.

Portions of the text have been adapted from several of my earlier publications; the permission of the publishers is gratefully acknowledged:

"Consensus by Committee: Philosophical, Social, and Political Aspects of Ethics Committees." In *The Concept of Consensus*, ed. K. Bayertz and H. T. Engelhardt, Jr. Dordrecht: D. Reidel Series in the Philosophy of Medicine, 1994.

"Ethics Consultation as Moral Engagement." *Bioethics* 5, 1 (1991): 44–56.

"Ethics by Committee: The Moral Authority of Consensus." *Journal of Medicine and Philosophy* 13 (1988): 411–32.

"Committees, Consensus, and Contracts." *Journal of Medicine and Philosophy* 16, 4 (1991): 393–408.

"What Means This Consensus? Ethics Committees and Philosophic Tradition." *Journal of Clinical Ethics* 1 (Spring 1990): 38–43.

Washington, D.C.   J. D. M.
August 1994

Contents

Introduction

This book stems from the confluence of two subjects that have interested me for the past ten years: the role of bioethics as a social institution and the nature of ethics panels, especially ethics committees. Both interests grew out of my evolution as a philosopher. Shortly after my arrival as a junior member of the Department of Philosophy at George Washington University in 1979, I was invited to participate in a multidisciplinary bioethics course. Although I had several friends in bioethics and had received some cursory exposure to the literature, this was my first formal experience with the field. I was impressed by the fact that students and practitioners from various disciplines were deeply interested in what a philosopher had to say about ethical issues in health care, something that was not necessarily true of my course offerings in more standard philosophical subjects. It was this opportunity to be part of a larger societal conversation that ultimately drew me away from the traditional academic philosopher's role and into medical education. I suspect that many other philosophers in bioethics have been attracted to the field for the same reason.

It struck me that bioethics is not only an academic pursuit but also a social movement in which philosophical ideas are, in a literal sense, vital. Perhaps this is inevitable in a "postmodern" society, a necessary search for something in which to believe in the face of technologically mediated death. What is more, the "aliveness" of philosophy in bioethical debates is combined with medical, legal, economic, and political considerations. When I began to study and participate in ethics committees, it seemed to me that sociology and social psychology also had to be added to the mix. It was in the context of ethics committees that I became curious about the moral status of consensus processes, though only much later did I appreciate that the bioethical project as a whole could be brought under this rubric.

Setting out to write a book about consensus in ethics committees, I found myself compelled to expand the study to ethics commissions, and saw finally the implications of a consensus orientation for the entire field of bioethics. Although some of the material might be considered an introduction to the field, especially chapter 2, I prefer to think of this book as a reintroduction to bioethics within a framework that incorporates resources from moral philosophy, political philosophy, the history of ideas, and the social sciences. My goal is to present a comprehensive account of moral consensus in bioethics in a liberal, democratic, pluralistic society.

During the five years that I spent writing this book, there was an explosion of interest in the subject of consensus. The source of this interest has mainly been the sense that American society today is less unified by a set of core values than ever before. The future of the republic, according to some commentators, rests largely on our ability to formulate a new public consensus about right and wrong. If this diagnosis of our current ills has merit, then bioethics is in the thick of the prescribed treatment. For modern bioethics treats subjects that are central to social action and to our conception of ourselves as human beings, subjects about which there is often no obvious consensus. Moreover, bioethics has become associated with a moral consensus about some features of physician-patient relations that is still rather novel. At the same time, in its short lifespan bioethics has also gained a remarkable degree of credibility. Whether this stature is deserved or not, it is another good reason to subject consensus processes in bioethics to careful study.

A different cause of the recent interest in consensus is the view that straightforward majority voting procedures (almost the only kind Americans are familiar with) do not always respect the legitimate interests of minorities. Other sorts of arrangements, such as weighted voting, have been suggested. Implicitly at least, bioethics has also been concerned with avoiding a rigid majoritarianism that strikes most people as inappropriate where sensitive personal values are at stake. Here again, from the standpoint of consensus processes, the way bioethics has gone about addressing specific issues has implications that go beyond bioethics itself.

This book is organized into chapters on empirical and conceptual aspects of moral consensus in bioethics. The first chapter is an orientation to the subject. Chapter 2 reviews the current state of the bioethical consensus in theory and practice and poses some impending problems within it. In chapter 3 I analyze the concept of consensus in philosophy and ethics, drawing a number of distinctions that will apply throughout the book and depreciating the usefulness of others. Chapter 4 reconstructs what I call the political rationale for the authority of moral con-

sensus in a liberal, democratic, and pluralistic society. Chapters 5 and 6 describe
the history and functions of ethics commissions and ethics committees, respec-
tively, and examine the consensus-related conceptual issues they raise. The experience with these ethics panels also suggests the practical limitations of the political rationale for the authority of moral consensus. In light of those limitations,
chapter 7 develops a philosophical account of the emergence of moral consensus
from ethically problematic situations, using an approach I call bioethical naturalism. In chapter 8 I explore philosophical models and social scientific theories of
small group processes. The final chapter assesses the implications of a consensus-
oriented account of bioethics, which I view as partly a social reform movement.

Deciding Together

1

The Challenge of Consensus for Bioethics

Consensus, expertise, and moral authority in the life sciences

- The chairperson of a hospital ethics committee instructs her colleagues about the importance of reaching consensus on the question of a patient's capacity to decline life-sustaining treatment.
- The members of a government commission render a set of recommendations that is believed to represent the society's consensus on the use of new genetic technologies.
- A newspaper headline announces that, according to the latest public opinion survey, consensus on abortion remains elusive.
- A task force of health care professionals develops a set of guidelines for the appropriate care of severely ill newborns which reflects the group's consensus.
- The director of a medical intensive care unit reminds her associates that the profession has an ancient consensus about the duty to preserve life.

Appeals to consensus are so common, and the relations embodied in consensus so ubiquitous, that we have become largely inured to them. One philosophical commentator has written that "[c]onsensus refers to types of relationships which may obtain between members of a society with respect to almost all their social activities and interactions."[1] The ubiquity of consensus in social relations, which has long been recognized by philosophers, is one thing. But consensus has also often been thought to have some intellectual merit, reaching an extreme in the ancient Roman concept of *consensus gentium*: that which is universal among men as the criterion of truth. In the modern world, and especially in diverse secular societies, the quest for consensus has achieved a nearly ritual status. Given the familiarity of this quest and the fact that consensus is commonly thought to help hold together our society's delicate fabric, consensus is a singularly important subject. Relatively neglected, however, is the rationale for reliance on consensus on *moral* issues, though in a liberal, democratic, pluralistic society there seems to be no practical alternative to consensus.[2]

This is a study of the nature, role, and significance of moral consensus in bioethics. "Bioethics" is a popular contraction for "biomedical ethics," which is the study of moral values in the life sciences and in their clinical applications. Bioethics, of course, has ancient roots in medical ethics, but in its current form this is a new field, scarcely thirty years old. Many reasons have been cited for the emergence of modern bioethics, including dramatic technical advances in the health sciences and a heightened awareness of individual rights.[3]

One characteristic of modern bioethics that distinguishes it from its historic precursors in medical ethics is a persistent skepticism about the moral authority of technical experts, whether that of the "bench researcher," the clinical investigator, or the attending physician. For example, laboratory scientists working on recombinant DNA technology or in the area of human genetics have been subjected to broad public scrutiny out of concern about "biohazards" in the first case and "playing God" in the latter case. The protocols of clinical researchers are subject to guidelines and to oversight whenever they involve the use of human or animal subjects. And clinicians are expected (at least in theory) to be as vigilant in guarding against "paternalistic" tendencies in relations with patients as they are about maintaining a level of competence in the treatment of patients.

Our skepticism that technical experts necessarily possess moral insight is not limited to those in the life sciences; in recent memory atomic physicists underwent a highly publicized period of criticism and self-criticism concerning the moral implications of their work. Nor are such doubts wholly new: Socrates famously derided the notion that those who are expert in one field must also be expert in another, let alone wise in a philosophical and moral sense. Yet this skepticism is not wholehearted, for even though we may have reservations about experts, we nevertheless admire them and reward them with perquisites that suggest they have a kind of wisdom. Scientists are granted the time and freedom to pursue their hypotheses, and most doctors enjoy relatively large incomes as well as a measure of public esteem. When scientists and physicians discuss social issues having to do with their fields, we are likely to give their views special attention, even if we do not automatically accept them.

Of course, those of us who are among the laity are in fact dependent on these experts throughout our lives, and especially during personal medical crises. Many questions central to bioethics involve moral and philosophical considerations but require a level of scientific knowledge: Is it worth the risk of creating new bacteria for agricultural purposes that could theoretically pose a threat to the ecosystem? Is an investigational drug a reasonable alternative to standard therapy for a cancer patient? Is cardiopulmonary resuscitation indicated for a stroke victim? The authority of experts in their fields is not always easy to disentangle from a more philosophical kind of insight.

The ongoing modern critique of technical expertise has not, therefore, led to casting it aside as irrelevant to moral insight, nor should it. Rather, it has engendered the widespread view that fields in which expert knowledge is power should be carefully monitored, as should the professional activities of their practitioners. Bioethics is one manifestation of this modern view with regard to the life sciences and their clinical applications. But if scientific expertise is not uncritically to be granted moral authority, some other human institution must act as a corrective. At certain times and places religious authority acting through ecclesiastical institutions has played this role. In secular and pluralistic societies such as ours, whatever common values there are that can form the basis for the polity also give societal consensus a perceived moral authority. Thus, in modern and "postmodern" societies it is that consensus rather than religious authority which constrains unbridled expert opinion on moral questions.

This is a highly democratic arrangement, for if consensus is the moral authority, then no one individual is. Whatever else consensus may be, it is surely a common or shared sense of things; therefore, in principle everyone is in a position to contribute. All may have a say, and since the scientist undeniably knows something important about the topic (though it is surprisingly hard to say exactly what that might be), he or she may well get a special hearing; but in theory there should be a group decision. To endorse consensus is not necessarily to endorse the idea of an explicit vote; indeed, some senses of the word *consensus* seem even to exclude the idea of a vote. For the most part, decision makers can rely on a sort of passive acceptance by the polity, especially concerning highly technical matters that do not excite immediate public interest. In other cases mere public acquiescence to a decision by some kind of leadership, although the most efficient form of consensus, may not be acceptable. Novel or controversial questions may require more deliberate consideration in a more public process, one that by common consent, or at least assent, is the soundest way to go about trying to achieve consensus.

But the history of consensus is no happier than the history of expertise. Taking the long view, Western culture on the whole is less confident about the authority of moral consensus than about that of moral expertise. Thus, the Western tradition tends to deny that consensus on *moral* questions has any validity in itself. Although there were of course prominent exceptions to this trend, such as the ancient Sophists ("Man is the measure of all things"), they are not usually celebrated as models of philosophical purity. Most of our venerated cultural figures, including Moses, Socrates, and Jesus, can easily be viewed as critics of moral

consensus. Indeed, the circumstances surrounding the deaths of all three have tra-
ditionally been attributed to the inherent moral failings of the mob, a powerful
brief against moral consensus

The institution of bioethics

Consensus processes have an important role in bioethics. This book is partly
motivated by the view that those processes have gone largely unappreciated and
unexamined. In general, the drastic change in medical ethics that has taken place
in the last three decades, from an acceptance of physician paternalism to an emphasis on patient self-determination, reflects an evolution in the consensus about
the essential nature of doctor-patient relations. In this trivial sense, any widespread
change in societal values can be regarded as a new consensus. Yet the processes
by which bioethics participates in the changing societal consensus about health
care present numerous nontrivial questions. Understood as a social institution,
bioethics is not only a field of study but also a set of social practices. As such, it
participates in the dominant social forms of its culture. In particular, as an institution it participates in the mechanisms that a diverse, liberal, democratic society
has devised to deal with uncertainty about moral concerns that arise in studying
the life sciences and in applying the knowledge that is gained from those studies.

To encourage or identify the development of consensus about novel and controversial issues, our society relies heavily on panels composed partly, but not
necessarily exclusively, of technical experts. Emerging questions of values in the
life sciences have been treated in the same way, and as a result experts in bioethics and related fields have been called on to contribute to panels concerned with
bioethical issues, both as members and as consultants. Since these panels operate
under a rubric that endorses consensus processes, both the institution of bioethics
and the individuals who are considered experts in the field have become closely
identified with consensus in the formulation of societal responses to ethical issues
in medicine and the life sciences. Interestingly, the life sciences have themselves
adopted the "consensus of expertise" model with regard to technical scientific
controversies as embodied in consensus conferences.[4]

Of course, bioethics as an academic field of study is only contingently related
to panels on social and ethical issues, for academic bioethics is not directly concerned with developing a societal response to these questions. It could be argued
that even academic bioethics makes some contribution to the development of such
a consensus, since all education presumably contributes to a society's conversation about its problems; but that is a fairly extended claim. Rather, the institution
of bioethics becomes involved in consensus panels, and thereby in consensus-
oriented deliberative processes, when its practitioners move out of the academic
setting and become members of or consultants to two types of organizations: governmental or professional policy-making bodies and institutions concerned with

the care of particular patients. In these ways consensus-oriented panels have become a part of the institution of bioethics. Furthermore, although bioethics as an academic subject is not directly engaged in the processes of achieving societal consensus, there is surely an iterative relationship between bioethics in the academy and bioethics in the policy-making and clinical realms. Bioethical theories and principles find their way into practice as well as teaching, and experience with bioethics in practice affects the way bioethical issues are conceptualized.

So far I have suggested that skepticism about the moral authority of technical experts in research and application of the life sciences has been accompanied by a growing role for consensus-oriented panels. It can hardly be denied that the institution of bioethics is rife with such bodies. Their internal consensus should be carefully distinguished from the wider social consensus about bioethical matters, even though they are often related. In this book I sort ethics panels into two general types: ethics commissions (hereafter referred to as commissions) and healthcare ethics committees (referred to as committees). The former category includes government bodies such as the National Commission for the Protection of Human Subjects of Biomedical and Behavioral Research, the President's Commission for the Study of Ethical Problems in Medicine and Biomedical and Behavioral Research, and the New York State Task Force on Life and the Law. It also includes groups empaneled by professional organizations for the specific purpose of examining novel or controversial bioethical problems that affect their fields, such as the panel on the ethics of fetal tissue research jointly sponsored by the American Fertility Society and the American College of Obstetricians and Gynecologists, or research groups created by academic organizations such as the Hastings Center. All of these panels tend to focus on matters of policy rather than on the care of individuals for whom they as institutions are responsible. Healthcare ethics committees, by contrast, concern themselves with issues affecting individuals for whose care the institution empaneling them is responsible. For the purposes of this book I consider that institutional review boards, infant care review committees, and healthcare ethics committees all fall into this category. Also in this group are the earlier kidney dialysis selection committees, or "God squads." Abortion selection committees and sterilization review committees, also earlier phenomena, are discussed in chapter 6 as precursors to ethics committees.

There is a certain kind of ethical review body that I do not include within either of these categories: the sort charged with peer review of professional misconduct. These bodies, whether appointed by professional organizations or under a legal jurisdiction, belong not to the institution of bioethics so much as to the institution of professional self-regulation. The matters with which they are concerned, such as a professional's sexual relations with patients or clients, are not bioethical issues in the usual sense because they are matters about which there is a relatively settled consensus. They are concerned with ethical "problems" in the sense that the actions they deal with are harmful to persons, but not in the sense that they present doubts about what conduct is morally preferable. This distinction is perhaps somewhat rough, but it is a common and, I think, a useful one. Often when the term *bio-ethics* is used in the literature, it is in contrast to these more traditional, garden variety ethical problems that have to do with grievous professional misconduct.

I consider both kinds of bioethics panels, commissions and committees, to be consensus-oriented in two important senses. First, they attempt to draw upon, articulate, and contribute to the emerging societal consensus on one or another bioethical issue. Second, their internal processes are mostly characterized by a desire to reach consensus within the group rather than to operate according to a parliamentary majority. Again, these are arguably iterative processes, since under certain circumstances the effort to achieve an internal consensus might be regarded as a miniature version of the debate taking place in the wider society.

The advent of bioethicists as public ethical experts who are themselves in search of consensus creates an interesting challenge for the field, expressed in part by Arthur Caplan:

The public face of bioethics makes Amcricans nervous because they hate ethical experts. And the people who are in the role of being called upon as experts are nervous because they know that without consensus about the foundations of the field, there may be a hole at the center of the enterprise.[5]

To augment the peculiarities of the situation Caplan describes, one might add that bioethicists themselves often have serious doubts about the moral authority of consensus, including their own, even while they depend on it. As intellectuals within the liberal and skeptical Western tradition, they are caught in the paradoxes that follow from the many senses of consensus. An example from the bioethical literature may serve to embody the paradoxical situation that Caplan describes. In an article on the need for research on ethics committees, two bioethicists complain that

little consensus exists about standards for education and skills necessary for membership on a committee, or for the internal operations of committees, for providing consultation as a committee member, or for procedural guidelines for the conduct of consultations.[6]

It is hard to deny that these are indeed important matters about which to achieve a consensus, especially given the growing popularity of these panels in health care. Yet on the same page, while commenting on a study of consensus among ethics consultants, the authors worry about an "unintended message" of this study "that ethics committees should always make a single consensus recommendation to resolve an ethical problem."[7] The assumption appears to be that expert consensus on standards for ethics committees is valid and desirable in a way that expert consensus on the assessment of a clinical ethics issue is not. We might be able to discern different senses of "consensus" operative in these observations, but they are also close enough to raise vital questions about the nature of a consensus in bioethics, if not to invite immense confusion.

The potential for confusion is also exemplified in a report by the Office of Technology Assessment on government ethics commissions. While warning about the dangers of "forced consensus" that can result from centralizing the formulation of bioethical policy and expressing doubts about the moral and political authority of consensus,[8] the report refers repeatedly to the "consensus" among its expert bioethics panelists about the optimal size of a commission, the merits of rotating membership, and the need for autonomy from the legislative and executive branches.[9] Again, while there is no inconsistency in these uses of a notoriously amorphous term, the fact that they can appear in such close proximity with very different implications indicates how badly needed is careful consideration of the different senses and of the various conceptual problems they carry with them.

The nexus of autonomy and consensus in bioethics

It is interesting to note that consensus-oriented panels assumed increasing importance in the institution of bioethics following the astonishing success of the patients' rights movement. The National Commission appeared hard on the heels of the decision in the *Quinlan* case, a milestone for patients' rights, and was itself closely followed by the proliferation of ethics committees and the establishment of the President's Commission. The movement to protect and promote patient autonomy has been closely associated with a trend toward consensus-oriented panels. Autonomy and consensus are both, in the first instance, political concepts; in fact, during the past two decades consensus-oriented commissions and committees have largely supported the movement toward autonomy for research subjects and patients.

If this observation has a paradoxical air, it is because autonomy and consensus are closely but ambiguously related. Bioethicists appreciate the importance of personal autonomy in our society's received liberal political philosophy, commonly expressed as "the consent of the governed." At several points in this book I argue that consensus *also* has an important place in liberal political philosophy, but one that has been somewhat obscured by the history of the idea of consensus and by a subtle but important shift toward the language of consent and away from that of consensus. When these tendencies are brought to light, it becomes clear that the nexus of autonomy and consensus is deeply woven in liberal political philosophy and in bioethics as well.

This nexus appears in political philosophy in the doctrine of "liberal neutrality," the view that, in a liberal society, the state should endorse no particular vision of the good life, but should instead provide a space within which men and women are free to strive for their own vision (autonomy), and to associate with others who share to some extent their vision of the good life (consensus). In a somewhat different sense of the terms, and at a logically prior level, the theory of liberal neutrality itself represents a consensus that individuals should be free to exercise their own autonomy. Although of enormous importance for modern civil society, the nexus of autonomy and consensus poses substantial challenges for bioethics, challenges that may in fact be insurmountable, for how can we hope to resolve problems such as whether doctors may assist in suicide if there are so many ideas about the purpose of life, or of reducing the waste of health care resources if there are so many ideas about what counts as waste?[10] Indeed, how can a society with so many different value systems, especially ethnic and religious ones, reach agreement about these kinds of issues? These are serious difficulties for a pluralistic society that is committed to a liberal political philosophy.

Traditional medical ethics largely codified ethical principles; unlike modern bioethics, it was not a forum for debate. But the issues characteristic of bioethics are, as it is often said, questions about which reasonable people might disagree. Yet there are in fact many propositions in contemporary bioethics on which there is a consensus, at least within the bioethical community. Liberal political philosophy, I will argue, has trouble authorizing consensus beyond the point at which it can be supported by settled principles. Yet the institutions of bioethics regularly seek to extend this more or less settled consensus into new ethical territory. How can these consensus-extending activities, typified by ethics panels, including commissions and committees, be authorized in a liberal society?

The answer lies partly in the qualities of the consensus-building processes themselves, and that requires a more frankly social scientific approach than has prevailed in most bioethical analysis. But before we can know what processes to examine, we need to appeal to social scientific theory for an enhanced understanding of the concepts involved. For example, philosophical writers tend to think of consensus as the result of an active decision-making process, perhaps engaged in by a group of abstract individuals, as in some models generated by social contract theory. Like so much bioethical and ethical theorizing, this understanding of consensus is sociologically naive. From a sociological standpoint, the greatest part of what counts as moral consensus is agreement by acquiescence, passive rather than active, and embedded in cultural traditions and interpersonal associations. This is one of the respects in which consensus is distinct from consent, for only the latter implies active, conscious agreement.

This suggests that bioethics should strive for an improved understanding of the dynamics of social life, an understanding that requires a close look at actual social practices. I call this approach the *naturalization* of bioethics. A naturalized understanding of bioethics by way of the study of consensus processes reveals a further common misconception, one that is represented in our ordinary language when we say that consensus is a "goal" to be "reached" or "achieved." Since consensus is a process as well as a goal, consensus judgments are bound up with the quality of the processes that led to that judgment. An improved understanding of consensus processes also helps us to distinguish consensus from compromise, with which it is often confused, with unfortunate consequences for an appreciation of the nature of ethical deliberation as a part of social life.

A goal of this book is thus to capture the significance of actual consensus processes for bioethics while not "reducing" moral philosophy to sociology. I think this can and must be done, for as bioethics becomes more and more engaged in societal decision making, greater pressure will be brought to bear upon it and its practitioners to retain a critical and independent moral position. Without it, bioethics will and should lose its credibility.

Consensus and bioethics

So far in this chapter I have been discussing the importance of consensus *in* bioethics; that is the focus of several chapters in this book. Since, as I contend, consensus is a subject of enormous importance in bioethics, it is also a subject of great moment *for* bioethics, in the sense that the nature of bioethics itself appears different once one adopts a consensus viewpoint. Yet writers in bioethics have had very little to say about consensus, and what they have had to say has often been either poorly informed or seriously confused.

Perhaps one reason why writers in bioethics have so little to say about consensus is that we are somewhat inured to it. Especially as compared to academic philosophy, much of the work in bioethics takes place in a collaborative mode with colleagues from other disciplines, including teaching and writing as well as working on commissions and committees. Another reason may be that modern academic bioethics was barely under way before its practitioners were in demand in the public arena, doing intellectual work that helped to influence the evolving consensus. Seen in this light rather than through the hackneyed and misleading framework of "theoretical" and "applied" ethics, the institution of bioethics is far more a part of evolving social forms than is generally appreciated. Surely it is more than an accident that, while bioethics was establishing itself as a field, some of the most exciting work in recent philosophy was seeking to rethink traditional problems in terms of moral discourse rather than moral knowledge. In that spirit, much of the burden of this book is to develop a conceptual framework in which bioethics is understood as grounded in actual social practices. If this aim can be achieved, it will be in part because, as usual, reality has outrun human understanding. Bioethics is already part of our society's moral discourse.

To understand both the role of consensus *in* bioethics and its importance *for* bioethics, I propose a pragmatic approach that I call bioethical naturalism. Resisting a simplistic fact-value dichotomy, bioethical naturalism takes actual moral experience as primary data for ethical inquiry. Moral experience includes, of course, the social dimension of ethical decision making as characterized by sociological and other sources. It also includes data from moral psychology that can help explain how moral consensus is possible from an individual as well as a social standpoint. Like any other experiential problem, moral uncertainty tends to stimulate a pattern of inquiry and represents an opportunity for a socially intelligent response. In short, bioethical naturalism recognizes that a novel moral consensus can proceed only from the intellectual and societal context in which we find ourselves, and that it must engage social processes. The "fit" between the social institution of bioethics and a naturalistic philosophical framework strikes me as inviting and important.

My pragmatic and naturalistic approach to consensus distinguishes me from those who, in the expression of the philosopher Nicholas Rescher, would "sanctify" consensus. For me, consensus is not a regulative ideal of human affairs, as it is for many European thinkers. I do not assume that consensus is a necessary goal of scientific inquiry or social relations, though in fact it often ends inquiry and sustains relationships. Rather, I take consensus to be a "lubricant" of the activities of men and women in civil society, something that is often but not always desirable. In this book I explore the implications of the fact that consensus is often unworthy in itself; that in our dominant political philosophy autonomy is a protection against the possibility of dictatorial consensus; and that there is a tendency toward consensus on moral values, a tendency that can be illuminated by the social sciences. In particular I urge that, while bioethicists need neither praise nor bury consensus in general, it behooves them to understand consensus processes because they are so much a part of the institution of bioethics.[11]

Consensus and controversy

Part of the success of bioethics lies in the fact that it is widely seen as a more or less neutral space in which social consensus processes can operate. In itself consensus is generally regarded as a highly desirable state of affairs, especially in a pluralistic society such as that of the United States. Evidence of the popularity of consensus is everywhere to be found in our public life, but one common manifestation is the frequency of appeals to consensus, particularly in relation to matters that are or could be controversial. Even the most subtle and challenging questions can be set aside to the extent that *some* consensus about them can be reported. In the public media a "lack of consensus" on this or that problem is bemoaned, while the prospect that consensus is within our grasp is celebrated. Scientific and technical discourse also marks the attainment of consensus as an important event. Indeed, one often has the feeling that, once consensus is announced by the appropriate individual or group, permission is implicitly given for mentation on the matter to cease. As the political scientist V. O. Key has written, "[T]he magic word 'consensus,' in short, solves many problems, but only infrequently is the term given any precise meaning."[12]

In a liberal and pluralistic society that emphasizes process resolution of controversies, this drive for consensus is understandable if not always admirable. A preoccupation with consensus for its own sake causes justifiable concern when it seems to preempt critical doubt. The Western philosophical tradition, as we shall see, is deeply divided in its attitude toward consensus.[13] On the one hand, it is highly skeptical about the tendency of consensus to thwart criticism and dissent; on the other hand, it relies on consensus to help strike the balance between individual self-expression and societal functioning. Moreover, at some point dissensus for its own sake can be as self-defeating as consensus for its own sake. One of the early philosophers of science, Charles S. Peirce, observed that in science, unlike in philosophy, inquiry about a matter ceases when there is no practical reason for further doubt. In many cases at least, consensus can thus be viewed as the appropriate conclusion of inquiry, and continuing criticism in those instances may be mischievous. But since inquiry is an open-ended affair, the method of science admits that any consensus is always tentative, and the matter may be reopened if and when a substantial basis for dissent emerges.[14]

The analogy between resolving scientific controversy and moral controversy is itself contentious, and I do not mean to beg the question of the relationship between fact and value, a subject to which I will return. For the time being it is enough to recognize that part of the ambiguity of the idea of consensus is that appeals to it are made in various contexts, including those of science, ethics, and social policy. In health care, for example, there are consensus conferences about technical medical questions and consensus-oriented processes about ethical issues. In both science and ethics consensus appears to be desirable because a majority vote seems somehow inappropriate. It is not easy to say exactly why this is so, though the intuition is strong and widely shared. Sometimes an ethics committee will reluctantly conclude that a vote must be taken; but if the motion passes only narrowly, the membership may decide not to take the authorized action after all. I have witnessed this result on several occasions. Out of a sense of the unseemliness of insisting on mechanical democratic processes when important moral values are involved, and from a desire to preserve the amity of the group, the majority is sometimes prepared, and even eager, to waive its privileges.

In the case of science a majority vote seems to be anathema, for science is conducted by experts who are supposed to have special access to the truth about their field of study. Since this access is presumably shared among them, it would be odd to think that a scientific question could be settled merely by finding out what more than half of the experts think. In particular, science is understood as governed by publicly observable demonstration rather than by personal opinion. Therefore, whatever is the truth of the matter should be available to all those with the appropriate expertise who have access to the evidence. Consensus is a way to preserve and protect this conception of the resolution of scientific questions, even though it is undoubtedly the case that there is often more disagreement among the experts than could be admitted by a straightforward notion of scientific consensus.

Superficially at least, consensus in ethics has a somewhat different appeal. The usual reluctance to subject ethical questions to a vote seems to stem from a sense that ethics should not be reduced to a simple matter of preference. But beyond this point there are different reasons to favor consensus. Thus, some believe that there are truths about moral questions just as there are truths about scientific questions, and that, like science, ethics cannot be governed by a majority view. For them, there is something discomfiting about voting on ethical issues; it seems tasteless or in some ill-defined way inappropriate to do so. Others worry about the "tyranny of the majority" and wish to protect those with sincerely held but nonconformist moral values from majority dictates, hoping that consensus will preserve a degree of flexibility in social relations. One manifestation of this flexibility may be a general decision to reach a "compromise."

Another similarity between consensus in science and in ethics is so elementary that it is easy to miss: consensus in either case is reached in a social context. To understand consensus processes fully requires the study of subjects proper to fields such as communications and small group theory. The study of consensus also comports with the recent growth of philosophical interest in the idea of community. Those who strive to find a middle ground between individualism and socialism often call themselves communitarians, emphasizing the importance of common interests and responsibilities as a basis for novel means to manage seemingly recalcitrant societal problems. I do not claim expertise in this philosophy, but the study of consensus is surely an important feature of communitarianism.

The relation between the ideas of community and consensus suggests a further and critical qualification of the idea of consensus. In the formulation of social and scientific policy there are familiar appeals to explicit and relatively formalized consensus processes; this is how both philosophers and policy analysts tend to think of consensus. But in the normal course of life consensus processes are informal and implicit. As the sociologist Manfred Stanley has written:

As against common meanings that are conscious in the minds of participants, there are also intersubjective meanings that are not necessarily consciously available in the subjective lives of most members of a population. Intersubjective meanings are constitutive assumptions that govern patterns of social practice. Any pattern of social practice can be regarded as grounded in beliefs, norms, and values that make that practice intellectually coherent. Consensus on such assumptions is not necessarily a matter of conscious agreement among participants in that social practice. Rather, it is a matter of indirect acquiescence expressed through simple willingness to engage in a given social practice.[15]

In behavioral terms, for the most part a broad public consensus is nothing more than a "disposition to acquiesce" in a certain way under certain conditions. My subsequent efforts to understand bioethics as a set of social practices, including the validation of moral consensus in terms of liberal political philosophy, rely on this more generous conception of consensus processes.

Scrutinizing bioethical consensus

All of the subjects I have mentioned so far bear on the way moral consensus manifests itself in bioethics. The Hippocratic and other medical traditions were concerned with moral as well as technical matters, and our own recent cultural memory retains the revealingly ambiguous idea of the "good doctor." If moral and technical concerns have always been tightly intertwined in medicine, so have moral and technical consensus. Indeed this must be the case, since the technical acts undertaken in the name of medicine have enormous moral implications.

Medicine surely does not require bioethics to achieve consensus, but bioethicists have succeeded in persuading physicians that their moral consensus will be more sound, or (and these alternatives do not exclude each other) that it will meet with more acceptance in the wider society, if bioethics has a hand in its formation. It is remarkable not only that medicine has opened to bioethics the inner sanctum of its fraternal ties but also that bioethics has achieved a level of social trust that medicine has lost. Up to now bioethicists have been perceived as mostly outside the system, disinterested critics who "watched the doctors."[16] Whether this popular perception has been true or not, it will be harder for the field to sustain it as both bioethics and its forms and practitioners become part of "the system" in various ways. Moreover, it is not always easy to differentiate between a consensus about an issue reached by the bioethical community, however that community is defined, and a bioethical consensus reached by the medical community or the general public. Since bioethical consensus has an influence well beyond the academy, the processes of achieving it demand scrutiny.

All of the themes discussed so far, and many more, are taken up in this book. The challenge that consensus presents to bioethics is manifold: What is the moral authority of consensus in a society such as ours? What are the best theories and arrangements for achieving moral consensus? To what extent are the institutions of the life sciences that bioethics studies themselves consensus oriented? How can disciplines not usually called on in bioethics, especially intellectual history and sociology, help bioethicists understand the processes of which they are a part? What contribution can bioethics make to enhancing prospects for the peaceful resolution of moral controversy in a pluralistic society? And what effect might answers to these questions, or even the very act of asking them, have on the way those who work in this field understand what they do?

Sometimes the speaker in parliamentary proceedings will seek the "sense of the house" on some matter. Often this occurs in lieu of a vote. Consensus decision-making processes are familiar in this context, where "the house" is the democratic assembly. Indeed, as I have noted, consensus processes are part of the very foundation of civil society in our Western democratic tradition and are by no means limited to representative bodies. Also, hospital denizens are familiar with old-fashioned expressions such as "the patient is in the house," or the term "house officer," which refers to the physician in postgraduate training.

Whether "the house" is the hearing room of a commission appointed by a governmental or professional authority or the conference room of a committee sanctioned by the professional staff or administration of a health care institution, bioethics is today no stranger to the scene. What it is doing there, what it can accomplish, how it may fail, and how it is in turn affected by its presence in such settings are questions long overdue for consideration.

Notes

1. Percy Herbert Partridge, *Consent and Consensus* (New York: Praeger Publishers, 1971), p. 73.
2. At least a passive consensus is necessary for some of the ground rules of a complex, modern society, a point that is pursued in chapter 4.
3. For a history of bioethics, see David J. Rothman, *Strangers at the Bedside: A History of How Law and Bioethics Transformed Medical Decision Making* (New York: Basic Books, 1991).
4. Robert M. Veatch, "Consensus of Expertise: The Role of Consensus of Experts in Formulating Public Policy and Estimating Facts," *Journal of Medicine and Philosophy* 16, 4 (1991): 427–46.
5. Arthur L. Caplan, "What Bioethics Brought to the Public," *Hastings Center Report*, Special Supplement, 23, 6 (1993): S15.
6. John C. Fletcher and Diane E. Hoffmann, "Ethics Committees: Time to Experiment with Standards," *Annals of Internal Medicine* 120, 4 (1994): 336.
7. Ibid., p. 336.
8. U.S. Congress, Office of Technology Assessment, *Biomedical Ethics in U.S. Public Policy: Background Paper*, OTA-BP-BBS-105 (Washington, D.C.: U.S. Government Printing Office, 1993), p. 27.
9. Ibid., pp. 35–36.
10. This question is also raised by Ezekiel J. Emanuel, *The Ends of Human Life: Medical Ethics in a Liberal Polity* (Cambridge, Mass.: Harvard University Press, 1991). Though I reach a different conclusion from Emanuel's, the issue is central to this book.
11. For a critique of extravagant claims for consensus, see Nicholas Rescher, *Pluralism: Against the Demand for Consensus* (New York: Oxford University Press, 1993). Rescher's foil is Jürgen Habermas, who argues that consensus is indispensable to communication. To a lesser extent he is also critical of John Rawls's social contract theory. Although I make use of some of the observations of Habermas and his followers in this book, I do not subscribe to their view of communication. And although I adopt some of Rawls's ideas, my notion of moral consensus according to the rationale of liberal political philosophy is hedged by concerns about small group processes. My idea of consensus is close to Rescher's middle way between consensus and dissensus, which he summarizes in four emphases that resonate with the account in this book: legitimate diversity, restrained dissonance, acquiescence in difference, and respect for the autonomy of others (p. 3).
12. V. O. Key, *Public Opinion and American Democracy* (New York: Knopf, 1961), p. 27.
13. Reference to *the* Western philosophical tradition is made advisedly, for it might well be argued that there is no single one. Indeed, my own account of moral consensus in bioethics relies on the fact that there is a historically important intellectual alternative, which in the eighteenth century manifested itself in the "moral sense" school. Still, few will deny that the tendencies to which I refer are central to the epistemological themes that characterize Western philosophy.

14. The locus classicus of this view is Charles S. Peirce, "The Fixation of Belief," in *The Collected Papers of Charles Sanders Peirce* (Cambridge, Mass.: Harvard University Press, 1931-35), S: 358–87.

15. Manfred Stanley, *The Technological Conscience*. (New York: Free Press, 1978), p. 102.

16. The phrase is from Albert R. Jonsen, "Watching the Doctor," *New England Journal of Medicine* 308, 25 (1983): 1531–35.

2

Consensus in Bioethics: Problems and Prospects

A new moral consensus

This chapter reviews various aspects of the current state of consensus in bioethics in three areas: clinical ethics, research ethics, and the ethics of health policy. In each case I rehearse what I take to be the contemporary consensus and offer examples of recent successes as well as continuing and emerging problems. In the chapters that follow I turn to case studies of moral consensus processes in bioethics and to philosophical and sociological aspects of that consensus. Naturally my emphases are influenced by my own professional experiences and interests. Nonetheless, it is useful to have at hand a characterization of the contemporary bioethical consensus. At the end of the chapter I briefly identify some likely future challenges.

So accustomed have we become to the bioethical consensus that this case analysis from a medical ethics textbook of the 1950s, before the advent of bioethics as a recognized field, may come as something of a shock. The case is titled "Concealing the Nature of His [*sic*] Disease from a Patient":

Miss A has chondrosarcoma. "Tell me," she pleads with Dr. B, "do I really have a cancer?" Dr. B, knowing that Miss A has ample time in which to prepare for death and wishing to spare her needless mental suffering, answers, "Your pains are due to arthritis."

Solution. If Miss A actually has arthritis, or if Dr. B is convinced that everyone at her age does have at least a mild case of arthritis, his answer is not morally wrong.

Explanation. Dr. B does not affirm that Miss A's pains are due *solely* to arthritis. If she does have arthritis even in a mild form, Dr. B is justified in thinking that her pain is due in part to the arthritis, and hence his answer is not a lie. If Miss A really wanted the entire truth, she would ask, "Are *all* my pains due to arthritis?" In such cases patients often do not wish to pursue the matter, preferring to accept an answer which leaves them with some ray of hope, even though in their hearts they may know what the facts are.[1]

After the theoretical work of the 1970s, clinical bioethics could hardly yield such a result. This example of a problem in truth telling goes to the very core of physican-patient relations. This much, then, seems uncontroversial: traditional medical ethics underwent a radical change under the influence of the new biomedical ethics. With rare exceptions, complete physician control over information and decision making, however beneficent the intent, is no longer in favor. Instead, physicians are, in theory, supposed to defer to patients in determining the goals of medical treatment.

Following from this fundamental shift are numerous examples of substantive guidance to physicians which have acquired the status of consensus views in the biomedical ethics literature. One is directly related to the case just cited: competent adult patients should be informed of their diagnosis unless it is certain that immediate and severe harm will result. Here are a few more, in no particular order: the competent adult patient is the one who should decide whether family members may also know the diagnosis; treatment decisions for cognitively impaired newborns should not be based simply on the fact of impairment; parents' religious beliefs should not present obstacles to providing life-sustaining treatment to their children; age is not in itself a basis for denying an adolescent the capacity to consent to treatment; there is a duty to treat AIDS patients, with suitable precautions; research with certain populations has inherently coercive potential; suffering should be alleviated even at the risk of hastening the dying process; elderly and dying patients should not routinely be restrained for administrative convenience; organs may be harvested from the deceased with the permission of the individual or of family members; there is no ethical difference between withholding and withdrawing life-sustaining treatment; neurological criteria are acceptable for determination of death; and so forth.

To say that these propositions are examples of bioethical consensus is not to say that there is unanimity about them. The idea that there is no ethical difference between withholding and withdrawing life-sustaining treatment, for instance, is one that at least some practicing physicians have a hard time accepting, whether their reasoning is sound or not. Yet, at least since the President's Commission reached this conclusion in the early 1980s, there has been no serious dissent from it among those recognized as bioethicists, and in their teaching it is a common point, albeit sometimes a provocative one.[2]

This is a random and unsystematic list, but it may perhaps serve as an orientation and preview. The next sections sketch the current state of consensus in bioethical theory and in the ethics of the clinic, the research setting, and health care policy. Readers steeped in bioethics will find some of this discussion elementary and may disagree with some of my constructions. But I hope to arrive at a relatively uncontroversial "report card" on the bioethics consensus as the field enters its fourth decade.

Consensus in bioethical theory

If there has been a consensus about bioethical methodology since the early 1970s, it has surely been that from various moral theories one can infer a discrete set of principles—autonomy, beneficence, nonmaleficence, and justice—and that these "midlevel" principles can in turn be applied to particular cases.[3] In terms of the foregoing discussion of levels of consensus, even if certain decision makers have identical preferences concerning the desired outcome of a particular case, they might well discover that, in spite of arriving at a common preference, they applied the principles a bit differently; or they might note differences in the moral theory or theories they selected to ground the principles. In spite of these theoretical limitations (if they are indeed limitations), this set of principles has become a convenient and practical schema around which most participants in bioethical debate have found they can rally.

The consensus that has formed around this approach to bioethical problems, like any consensus, has intellectual and sociological sources of legitimacy. Intellectually, this set of principles includes certain critical elements: some are historical (the Hippocratic emphasis on doing no harm); some are philosophical (the idea of justice as fairness); and some are legal (the concept of bodily integrity). Other sources of the bioethical consensus are more sociological in nature: in a pluralistic society with a powerful medical profession, a conceptual scheme that strives to "balance" personal autonomy with professional beneficence is quite desirable. Other sources for the consensus are still more specific; certain influential writers have published treatises that provide a secular methodology that bioethics had been lacking.

In practice these bioethical principles are not usually themselves subject to much attention, save among the abstract theorists. Instead, the principles are normally offered to clinicians and students as "guidelines" that can help to give order to a morally disorienting state of affairs. The principles are therefore the beneficiaries of a presumed consensus, though often as discussion proceeds, the participants realize that significantly different weighting of the principles may follow from different moral theories. Still, anyone who has ever worked through an actual clinical case with a group of anxious health care providers appreciates the availability of the "bioethics mantra": autonomy, beneficence, nonmaleficence, justice.

The regnant emphasis on principles in bioethics has received increasing criticism lately, which has come from several directions. Arguments have been advanced that principles are either too broad or too narrow. The former position is taken by those who advocate a case-based or casuistic approach,[4] while the latter is taken by those who advocate a unified theoretical approach.[5] In general, these critics of principlism in bioethics argue that the mere recitation of principles divorced from actual cases and not framed by a moral theory is on the one hand arid and on the other groundless.

Thus, the proponents of a modern casuistry urge that the moral life in all its richness can emerge only from a wide variety of actual situations. Although principlists may think of their principles as being in reflective equilibrium with experience derived from cases, casuists seem to think that the bioethics mantra has acquired a nearly axiomatic life of its own. Rather than an ethical system that applies principles to cases "from the top down," they argue that in practice principles emerge through experience with real cases, or "from the bottom up." There are various techniques in the art of casuistry, but vigorous use of analogy is among the most important. For example, by starting with paradigmatic exemplifications of certain common precepts or maxims (viz., "Don't kick a good man when he's down"), the elements of the paradigm case can be systematically varied until one discerns which are its essential features, without which a case would fail to satisfy the maxim.

For those interested in the development of moral consensus, the casuistic approach has its attractions. An ethics committee could reflect on a number of historic cases, both from its own institution and from others, and array them on a continuum according to the degree to which their outcomes satisfied some particular maxim. When considering future cases, the members would be prepared to identify the crucial elements that distinguish them from the paradigm cases. Consensus on the case at hand should flow from this process.

In assessing the "new casuistry" in bioethics, John Arras notes the ambiguous role played by theory. Sometimes the new casuists seem prepared to latch on to any source of moral guidance that happens to be lying around, while at other times they appear to give pride of place to moral theories devised by academic philosophers. Appealing as the notion of a "case-by-case" ethics might be, particularly when one wants to avoid higher-level philosophical contention, Arras concludes that casuistry is a method that is perhaps modest in its theoretical commitments, but does not entirely eschew theory.[6]

Insisting on consensus on a particular moral theory has been by far the least popular option in bioethics. In fact, it might not be hyperbolic to assert that one of the features that has distinguished moral philosophy and applied ethics has been the latter's rejection of the hegemony of any single theory. After all, it was the very effort to develop an analytic "metaethics" to adjudicate among the moral theories that led finally to the widely recognized aridity of Anglo-American moral philosophy by the 1960s. These conditions finally gave rise to applied ethics and to a renewed interest in normative questions. Moreover, the idea that a single moral theory can be applied, in deductive-nomological fashion, to specific practical ethical problems is commonly derided in bioethics as an "engineering" approach. But the critics of principlism call attention to the shortcomings of a bioethics that lacks a comprehensive theory, whether based on potentially conflicting principles or on intrinsically inconclusive cases.

A different sort of critique of the standard methodology which evokes principles in bioethics comes from feminist writers such as Susan Sherwin.[7] The feminist focus is not on the breadth or narrowness of the principles but rather on the very idea of using principles in addressing human problems. The use of a "disciplined," rule-oriented approach is taken as an example of a rigid, "masculinized" thinking which obscures the fact that one's native human sympathies will (and should) have a great deal to do with one's conclusion. Rather than preoccupy ourselves with principles and rules, according to this position, it would be better to look to procedures that will yield the arrangement that is most satisfactory to all those who stand to gain or lose by the outcome. Instead of wielding lawlike regulations in a "masculine" attempt to dominate what must remain unruly situations involving real pain and loss, we should find a way to bring everyone together in as sensitive and humane a manner as the situation allows.

The feminist critique of procedures based on fixed principles or rules remains unsatisfactory to many. Some find it anarchic or unrealistic; others regard it as irrelevant to most substantive bioethical issues. For our purposes, what is particularly interesting about the feminist critique is that it endorses a case-by-case consensus that looks directly to the protagonists in a particular state of affairs rather than to abstract principles from which a solution is then derived. In this respect, feminism urges a more intimate and personal quest for consensus.

The informed consent consensus

Clinical ethical conflicts are occasions for crafting the consensus that must emerge in this era of new relations between doctors and patients. In the example that follows, I hope to indicate some of the ways in which these conflicts express themselves within the procedural consensus that is being developed and highlight some of the limitations of that consensus—limitations that are especially challenging to ethics committees as they try to work within and advance the emerging consensus. Readers familiar with contemporary clinical ethics will recognize the issues raised and the conclusions drawn in the scenario.

Ms. A is a seventy-two-year-old widow who lives alone. After undergoing a stroke at home, she manages to telephone for help. A previous such episode two years ago left her partially disabled. When she arrives at the emergency room she is unconscious, and her respiratory drive is dangerously low. She is intubated and admitted to the intensive care unit. While Ms. A is in the ER, her daughter, who is her only adult child and who has been helping to take care of her, arrives and protests that her mother wishes no further life-sustaining measures. "She only wanted to be taken to the hospital so she could be kept comfortable in case she survived," her daughter says. "I showed the doctors that I had my mother's durable power-of-attorney and her living will, but they still went ahead and did what they did." The living will states that Ms. A wants no artificial life support should she become irreversibly unconscious. The durable power of attorney empowers her daughter to make all medical decisions for her should she be deemed incompetent. Twenty-four hours after her stroke, Ms. A is at best minimally conscious, unable to respond to queries about her wishes. Her daughter insists that she be extubated at once, in accordance with Ms. A's advance directives. Nursing notes during this first day of hospitalization indicate that Ms. A's daughter has occupied inordinate amounts of staff time with her constant complaints about her mother's situation.

There are a number of elements of such a case which must be separated. First, there is a consensus that patients in life-threatening situations must be treated unless there has been time to ascertain their wishes to the contrary. Since Ms. A called 911, the emergency medical team was obligated to institute life-saving procedures if they were not in good faith comfortable with the information they had about any wishes to the contrary. In practice, it is highly unlikely that emergency personnel would make such a judgment under these circumstances, especially since they are not trained to do so: "code and treat" is the first rule of emergency medicine. Although some jurisdictions have created out-of-hospital "do-not-resuscitate" orders, these instances are still highly exceptional.

Second, like the emergency medical technicians, an emergency room physician who is insecure about the medicolegal status of documents and transfers of decision-making authority would be most unlikely to violate the first rule of emergency medicine, which is to represent the expert view of the patient's best medical interests. The social consensus at this point in the story is somewhat less clear since there is a conflict between the dictum of erring on the side of life and that of respecting a patient's preferences, both of which values are incorporated into most living will legislation. The question here is, what level of evidence of patient preferences should be required when life hangs in the balance?

Third, were Ms. A competent, she would have every legal and (according to the secular moral consensus on medical ethics) moral right to insist that no further treatment be introduced. On this there is a broad social consensus and an acceptance, albeit sometimes a grudging one, by the medical profession. She would have the right to insist on removal of the ventilator, though this is still met with resistance by a few recalcitrant physicians who see the withdrawal of life support as active euthanasia, an interpretation most bioethicists would consider erroneous.

Fourth, a patient's advance directives are normally to be accorded the same weight as if she were currently insisting that her wishes be respected, whether those wishes are substantive (viz., "I do not want X") or procedural (viz., "I want B to decide for me"). To fail to honor these directives is to place a third party (other than the patient or her designated agent) in the role of decision maker for the patient, thus pushing the problem back a step, for then it is that person's values that will determine what is done to the patient. For their part, Ms. A's physicians have made it clear that their preference would be to wait another two or three days to assess the trajectory of her progress, in the hope that she will become lucid enough to express her current wishes.

Fifth, the advance treatment directives present an interesting problem. On the one hand, Ms. A's substantive directive specifies a condition for removal of life support—permanent loss of consciousness—which does not apply to her at this point within a reasonable range of medical certainty. On the other hand, her daughter is legally empowered to speak for her; and even without legal empowerment, as the closest living relative she would have been the presumptive surrogate. But the daughter wants to go further than the living will specifies. When this discrepancy is pointed out to the daughter (who is no slouch), she responds that the living will does not say that artificial life supports are to be removed *only* if her mother is permanently unconscious. Thus, she argues, the living will is irrelevant right now, and she is the only proper decision maker for her mother.

To this discussion I should add the observation that feminists would point out: that as women, both Ms. A and her daughter are vulnerable to the (male) assumption that they don't know what they want, and thus their protestations against aggressive treatment are liable to be taken less seriously than would be the case if they were men.[8]

This sort of scenario, with medical, moral, legal, psychosocial, and administrative elements, is an example of how the new era of doctor-patient relations has led to novel issues that often find themselves on the agenda of ethics committees. In such cases there is a temptation to view the problem as a legal one *simpliciter*, especially since the problem seems to be one of the priority of one legal document or another. But it is not always practical or desirable to take every such case to court, though it may be necessary if no accommodation can be worked out.

The specific problem facing the parties in the case of Ms. A emerges in a highly sophisticated and articulate framework of moral consensus about the issues at stake. This is in itself remarkable, considering how little of this framework existed or was accepted by our social institutions even two decades ago. The new medical ethics, embodied in the doctrine of informed consent, has achieved this rapid acceptance because it is part of the modern liberal paradigm of procedural consensus on moral issues. This is reflected in the law, in which a clear consensus has emerged concerning at least the ethical issue of forgoing life-sustaining treatment. Alan Meisel has described and traced the roots of the legal consensus, beginning with *Quinlan* in 1976 and culminating in *Cruzan* in 1990. The specific points are important enough to be quoted verbatim:

1. Competent patients have a common-law and constitutional right to refuse treatment.

2. Incompetent patients have the same rights as competent patients; however, the manner in which these rights are exercised is, of necessity, different.
3. No right is absolute, and limitations are imposed on the right to refuse treatment by societal interests.
4. The decisionmaking process should generally occur in the clinical setting without recourse to the courts.
5. In making decisions for incompetent patients, surrogate decisionmakers should apply, in descending order of preference, the subjective standard, the substituted judgment standard, and the best interest standard.
6. In ascertaining an incompetent patient's preferences, the attending physician and surrogate may rely on a patient's "advance directive."
7. Artificial nutrition and hydration medical treatment and may be withheld or withdrawn under the same conditions as any other form of medical treatment.
8. Active euthanasia and assisted suicide are morally and legally distinct from forgoing life-sustaining treatment.[9]

Of more interest for the purposes of this study than Meisel's lawyerly defense of his formulation of the consensus is his account of the evolution of consensus in the legal system. As he points out, and as I have noted, consensus need not represent unanimity. In the legal system such consensus would be hard to achieve, owing to the multiplicity of jurisdictions (all the states, the District of Columbia, Puerto Rico, and the territories), and the fact that most have not heard an appellate right-to-die case. There are also differences between state legislative statutes on advance directives. In the state courts there is a tendency for appellate judges to look to other jurisdictions that have a record of persuasive argument in certain areas. This is true of the New Jersey Supreme Court on right-to-die cases since *Quinlan*, for example, but not of the New York Court of Appeals, which has been on the fringe of the legal consensus on this subject.

It is important to note that there are also less formal lawmaking processes that include the interaction between law and clinical practice. Meisel notes that very few cases on forgoing life-sustaining treatment are ever litigated, even though in clinical practice this occurs with some frequency. The fact that the decision to forgo such treatment is well accepted clinically has an important effect on the law's willingness to countenance the practice under certain circumstances. The policy statements of professional organizations in health care have also had an effect on the law.

Beyond informed consent

Informed consent has a settled character that little of the rest of bioethics enjoys. If we vary the case a bit, another implication of the new medical ethics surfaces. Imagine that another patient, this one in a well-documented persistent vegetative state, is represented by a duly appointed surrogate who insists that the patient be placed on dialysis for her kidney disease. Informed consent doctrine does not cover this sort of case, for it does not posit a blanket entitlement to services; rather, this scenario seems more to be a problem involving the limits of consumer choice in health care. Furthermore, although it is a crucial point of reference, informed consent by no means presents a recipe for the moral management of all cases.

As H. Tristram Engelhardt, Jr., has observed, the informed consent doctrine promoted by biomedical ethics is a virtual lingua franca of modernity.[10] In classical liberal terms, respect for individual self-determination is the very condition for civil society, for entrance into the social contract. The bioethical consensus that has grown up around the doctrine of informed consent in health care is really a reflexive confirmation of our society's essential philosophy: the answer to the "who should decide?" problem is that everyone should decide for himself or herself, under conditions of freedom and equality. Thus, Adam Smith's concept of the invisible economic hand is also useful in the moral realm. That is, on the whole, the superior moral arrangement for a society is that in which each member is able to function as a moral agent concerning his or her own plan of life.

Now, consider how this procedural consensus is applied to those who, unlike Ms. A, have left no advance directives. At the bedside the absence of a substantive social consensus on decision making for the noncompetent patient who has left no advance directives leaves those decisions in the hands of an assortment of advocates, usually some combination of close relatives and health care providers. It is this small group that must reach agreement on a course of treatment or nontreatment, and in this respect contemporary medicine is not very different from its historic antecedents. Some states have tried to regulate the environment of substantive decision making for noncompetents whose prior wishes are unknown by requiring their surrogates to choose according to the patient's best interests. But what is the moral authority of the substantive "microconsensus" arrived at by family and physicians for a patient whose life hangs in the balance? How does its justification compare to that of the established procedural social consensus?

To some extent the latter question has already been addressed. If the bioethical doctrine of informed consent is a validation of the liberal social consensus, then at least it applies in exactly the same fashion to everyone. But individuals for whom life-or-death decisions must be made represent a wide variety of circumstances, both medical and personal. Furthermore, responsibility for these decisions is necessarily spread unevenly throughout the society, falling mainly on the patient's family (usually the female members, who tend to be the uncompensated care givers) and physicians. Therefore, any particular decision on behalf of the noncompetent patient is often subject to more doubt than the generalization that each competent adult should decide for himself or herself, come what may.

Yet the reality of our pluralistic society is such that we have to live with a less than wholly satisfactory solution to the problem of deciding for others, for given a diversity of values, we can reach no detailed substantive consensus on treatment for the seriously ill. Hence, the contemporary battleground in clinical decision making is laid out precisely between those parties who have the strongest claim to speak for the noncompetent patient without advance directives: physicians and families. In whose favor should the social consensus be decided? What guidance do the liberal values of freedom and equality provide?

On occasion relatives or close friends of those who are incapable of speaking for themselves and who have dissented from the decisions of health care professionals have been obliged to go to court for relief. There are increasing signs that the presumption in favor of professional authority may be shifting somewhat. The husband of a New York woman who was aggressively treated at the end of her life against his wishes argued that he should be relieved of paying the bill, totaling $100,000, because the services were unwanted. His position failed, but on technical grounds.[11] Strenuous arguments have been presented in the legal literature that the burden of proof concerning appropriate treatment should be shifted from those who know the patient best, generally the family, to the institution.[12] And many well-publicized cases of conflict between families and institutions have led hospitals to try to find new ways to accommodate a family's views about a patient's true wishes. Even this will not be a universal solution. As studies of surrogate decision making have documented, families as traditionally conceived are often not the best guide to a patient's wishes.[13] This lesson has been learned in the AIDS era, when physicians sometimes call on patients' close friends rather than biological relatives to assist in decision making. Families are increasingly coming to be defined in terms of social intimacy rather than bloodlines.

Still more troubling are cases involving individuals who are "moral strangers" to those responsible for their care. Those whose preferences cannot be known and whose interests are highly ambiguous, such as the very young, those with profound cognitive impairments, and those who are incapacitated and without social connections, are indeed "limit cases" for a clinical ethics founded on self-determination and beneficence. The doctrine of substituted judgment, devised by courts as a way of deciding for such individuals, depends on a fictional role reversal and has been rightly criticized. In particular Robert Weir has argued persuasively that the courts should drop the fiction of substituted judgment in favor of a frank best interests standard.[14] Those who are now competent and those who were once competent and whose preferences can be discerned should simply have their preferences respected, so that even in the latter case reference to substituted judgment is redundant at best.

Surely there will and should be continued debate about the most appropriate ethical standard to be applied to moral strangers. Given the vulnerability of human beings in this position, the fact that this question is unsettled is itself an expression of respect for them, for it indicates how seriously their interests are taken. There are some important matters about which we might not wish for a settled consensus, and the ethics of medical treatment for moral strangers is one, in spite of the difficulties this creates for those charged with their care. More generally, it would be odd to depreciate the consensus concerning patient self-determination because it fails to provide satisfactory guidance for the treatment of patients whose preferences are a matter of speculation. By the same token, this central doctrine of the modern medical ethics consensus should not be forced into a role it cannot play.

Before we leave this subject, it is worth noting that some data are available concerning the consensus among ethics consultants on their likely recommendations in certain sorts of cases. Ellen Fox and Carol Stocking surveyed 154 ethics consultants for their reactions to a case of a patient in a persistent vegetative state receiving artificially administered food and fluids. Of various scenarios in which nontreatment was an option, the one that stipulated that the patient had left an advance directive declining life-prolonging treatment and that the patient's family wanted this treatment to cease was the only one in which the consultants were in general agreement (87 percent) not to treat. The other scenarios varied the patient's wishes and those of the family, and none of them received more than 50 percent agreement to stop treatment.[15] While it is perhaps surprising that there was no consensus about the other scenarios, it is worth remarking on the high degree of agreement on one of them. As the authors of the study observe:

Considering the prevailing attitudes of only a few years ago, when ethicists hotly debated whether denying food and fluid was ever permissible, the finding that general agreement now exists in this area is remarkable in itself.[16]

The research ethics consensus

The moral consensus on the use of human beings in biomedical research is in some respects more settled than that concerning patients in nonresearch settings. For example, it is largely agreed that informed consent requirements should be even more rigorous in research because of the absence of reliable direct benefits to participation for the human subject. (There may, of course, be indirect benefits to participation, such as the satisfaction of helping others.) Although the reasonableness of this moral consensus may appear transparent to most contemporary readers, research ethics has undergone a profound evolution in the twentieth century. Nazi abuses of human beings during the Holocaust and a series of highly publicized incidents in the United States and elsewhere, some of them involving well-meaning investigators, have led to a far more cautious approach toward research on human subjects than that which prevailed decades ago. The very idea of using humans as means to further ends rather than as ends in themselves, the essence of their role in research, is contrary to a widely accepted philosophical maxim. It is hardly irrational to contend that no one should be exposed to unnecessary risk in the name of science. But in our society we have in effect concluded that research involving human subjects should go forward when participation is voluntary; the risk appears to be minimal; and the foreseeable benefits to others, if not necessarily the subject, are substantial.

Even under these conditions the participation of children, who are incapable of giving fully informed consent, has been regarded by some (most famously Paul Ramsey),[17] as unacceptable. Indeed, it is in the case of pediatric research that the "utilitarian" basis of the research ethics consensus is most obvious, for it is large numbers of other children who will most likely benefit from the investigational drug or device rather than the relatively few young subjects. Thus, special additional constraints have been placed on pediatric research, including in particular the standard that children should not be exposed to any more risk than is associated with a "minor increment over minimal risk," where minimal risk is defined as that associated with the child's daily activities or a routine physical examination.[18]

There are, of course, a number of loose threads within this rather settled consensus. For instance, although it is common to distinguish between therapeutic and nontherapeutic research, it is not always easy to tell the difference. As I have noted, research participation may be of benefit to the subject apart from any advantages directly associated with the drug or device being tried, such as closer attention by more health care professionals. Furthermore, as Robert Levine has pointed out, a placebo-controlled trial of a drug expected to be beneficial will not help the control group; is the research then "therapeutic" or not?[19] Periodically there is renewed discussion about the extent to which prisoners or college students are truly able to give uncoerced consent to research participation. These, however, are not the aspects of the research ethics consensus that have been subject to the greatest dispute in recent years.

Research ethics and women of reproductive age

In the early 1960s the drug thalidomide was prescribed to many pregnant women to help prevent nausea. It was especially popular in Scandanavia, but a suspicious Food and Drug Administration (FDA) official held up approval in the United States. When many of the children were subsequently born with foreshortened limbs, it became clear that thalidomide was indeed highly teratogenic. This experience and others helped create grave concern about exposing pregnant women to new drugs, a concern that was adopted by the research community. Pharmaceutical manufacturers reacted as well to worries about legal liability. There were not only ethical and legal but also methodological elements to this consensus. The hormonal cycles of women from menses to menopause affect the ways they metabolize drugs, thus creating variables for which corrections would have to be made, potentially increasing the costs of research. Gradually not only pregnant women but also all women of reproductive age came to be viewed by implicit consensus as largely barred from participation as subjects in drug studies, including clinical trials.[20]

Like so many ethical views this one seemed wholly reasonable until new considerations and circumstances subjected it to reexamination. By the mid-1980s it had become apparent that relatively little is known about the effects of major medications on women. Advocates for women and political leaders pointed out that certain drug studies, including a large-scale study of the effects of aspirin on the prevention of heart disease, were performed wholly on men, but the results were then generalized to women. As a result, physicians are required to do more guesswork about appropriate dosages in women than in most of their male patients. Moreover, in this country most drugs are prescribed to women, many of whom are in their reproductive years. Furthermore, the AIDS epidemic called attention to the role of perinatal transmission of HIV, the virus that causes AIDS, and to the need to do research with HIV-positive pregnant women in order to determine the possibilities of blocking transmission to a fetus.[21]

In light of these and other developments, federal agencies were under increasing pressure to reassess their position on women of reproductive age in clinical studies. In 1993 the National Institutes of Health formed a Task Force on the Recruitment and Retention of Women of Reproductive Age in Clinical Trials, of which I was a member. The NIH also contracted with the Institute of Medicine (IOM) of the National Academy of Sciences to examine the specific ethical and legal obstacles involved in recruiting women into clinical trials, a project for which I was also a consultant. In a bit of remarkable timing, during the IOM committee's workshop on this subject, the FDA announced that it was revising its 1977 guidelines on this matter, which embodied the previous consensus on the participation of female subjects. The new guidelines, it was announced, would require the involvement of nonpregnant women in virtually all phases of federally funded drug research. The NIH had revised its policy somewhat earlier, but the FDA's shift on the matter was especially significant from the standpoint of the approval process for new medications.

Thus, in a very short time what seemed an obvious protection for a "vulnerable" population, women of reproductive age and their possible children, came to be viewed as an overly restrictive standard that prevented women from receiving the same quality of medical care as men. In a word, the policy appeared to be exclusionary rather than protectionist. To be sure, this was partly a result of a more general shift in attitudes toward restrictive drug approval which emerged from the AIDS era, as well as the influence of feminism finally being felt at the highest levels of the research establishment. To many commentators, one of the most objectionable aspects of the historic policy has been a persistent characterization of male physiology as normal or standard, from which reference point female physiology is deviant. Indeed, one of the great ironies of traditional research practices may be a tendency to overestimate the risks of research to female germ cells and underestimate the risks to male germ cells. The latter are known to be vulnerable to numerous mutagens from industrial as well as pharmaceutical sources, but this consideration has not resulted in widespread ethical or legal worry about males of reproductive age in clinical studies and trials.

Moral consensus and health care policy

In comparison with clinical and research ethics, it is more difficult to identify substantive propositions about which modern bioethics has reached consensus concerning health care policy. Many moral issues at the policy level have to do with the allocation of scarce or expensive resources; in philosophical parlance, they involve problems of distributive justice. On certain policy matters, however, there is appreciable consensus. For example, in the field of organ distribution arrangements between donors and recipients engineered by private physicians are no longer thought to be acceptable. Organs are to be distributed by means of a public system based on "objective" medical criteria such as severity of illness, according to the philosophy that organs should be treated as gifts rather than as commodities, and that waiting time should be a factor in allocation. In the ethics of public health, draconian measures such as quarantine and confinement for the control of infectious disease are no longer presumed to be appropriate; instead, transmission mechanisms and civil liberties considerations must be factored into a comprehensive policy.[22] Finally, the ethics of research on human subjects is closely tied to health policy and is part of the groundwork of modern bioethics.

Yet modern bioethics has failed to generate a consensus on access to health care, and in particular on the question whether there is a moral right to a minimal level of care. Later in this book I will review the President's Commission's internal struggles on this issue, which were emblematic of social uncertainty on the matter. If the rhetoric of the "right to health care" has reemerged in this country, that is not because the philosophical debate of the 1970s and early 1980s has been re-solved. Rather, it is because the continuing increases in the cost of health care, and the inability of so many Americans to attain adequate health insurance, or any at all, has finally made the issue politically impossible to ignore. Business leaders have been especially concerned about the effects of our employment-based system on their ability to compete in international markets. In this case the market appears to have succeeded in creating a moral consensus (or at least a consensus with moral implications) where philosophical discussion could not.

Nonetheless, although the debate about access is terribly important in health care policy, the failure to achieve a bioethical consensus seems the exception rather than the rule, seen alongside other achievements in this area. Still, it is an impor-tant exception, and it would be useful to find some explanation for this state of affairs. One common explanation is that American society has clung to a rights-oriented philosophy of health care distribution. That portion of the liberal tradi-tion that emphasizes individual entitlements (the labor theory of value being a typical doctrine) fits well with a classic market. But modern health care services are not such a market because they involve the aggregation of social wealth, both public and private, in large pools of capital. Thus, unlike in traditional exchange relations, my access to a CAT scanner is not simply a matter of my being able to pay for the service, whether out of pocket or through an insurance premium, for the service would not exist if not for the social investment in development, production, and distribution of the device. Under these circumstances, it may be argued, communitarian values are better suited than market values to modern health care.

As a complement to this analysis I would offer an account that emphasizes consensus processes rather than philosophical views. Unlike all or nearly all of the other issues I have mentioned, the debate over access to health care requires the active engagement of many sectors of society and of all those groups that participate in financing health care delivery. By contrast, most of the bioethical issues about which consensus has been reached have been amenable to deliberation and negotiation within a far smaller group of experts and opinion leaders, usually followed by acquiescence on the part of the general public. Thus, the sheer political complexity involved in reaching consensus about what is owed to all Americans in terms of health care weighed heavily against achieving any widely acceptable formulation—this will continue to be the case unless the financial burdens of continued inaction become even more unacceptable.

Ethics and cost constraints in health care policy

Whatever institutional shape the new interest in health care rights ultimately takes, three goals will continue to dominate the conversation: access, cost containment, and quality of health care. The first goal apparently requires coordinated public action, and is being debated at the federal level. Whatever the ultimate result, costs must be contained while the provision of quality care is assured. The most popular, if still controversial, proposal to accomplish these goals is called managed health care. A Nixon administration initiative in the early 1970s called for the expansion of enrollment in the pioneer managed health care firms, health maintenance organizations. Today millions of people are enrolled in HMOs or other types of managed health care plans. Although these do not yet dominate the landscape of health care distribution, a consensus seems to be forming that some of their essential elements will be part of any future system.

Managed care organizations or health plans are both insurers and providers of health care. In order to meet their goals, health plans monitor the practice of their physicians and other clinicians. They attempt to ensure that enrollees are not subjected to more tests and procedures than are indicated. This is done by reversing the traditional financial incentives for the providers: instead of incentives to overtest and overtreat, as in fee-for-service practice, there are incentives to undertest and undertreat. These incentives take various forms but often have to do with a bonus pool that is larger if there are minimal levels of test ordering and referrals to specialists. These arrangements are shocking in contrast with the traditional ones only if one is naive about the consequences of too much medical attention for patients. Gail Povar and I have argued that, as providers as well as insurers, managed care plans acquire the moral obligations of health care agents toward their patients, including that of making a minimal level of skill available to all patients and serving as an advocate for all patients.[23]

My purpose is not to explain all the intricacies of managed care or to engage in a lengthy discussion of managed care ethics, but to suggest that a new consensus may be forming around a value that has not been at the core of writings on doctor-patient relations. Simply put, the new medical ethics that emphasize patient autonomy as a counterweight to physician beneficence is being further ramified by the value of justice toward all members of the health plan.[24] Under these conditions, both the provider and the enrollee have certain obligations not to overuse resources that are the common property of all who have invested in the plan. If we are in the midst of an emerging consensus that there are indeed such obligations, then this amounts to as profound a change in society's understanding of physician-patient relations as the advent of "shared decision making." But a managed health care consensus can succeed only if trusting relations between doctors and patients are preserved, regardless of the way doctors are reimbursed. All the more important, then, that the ethics of managed care receive ongoing attention.

Continuing challenges for consensus in bioethics

Thus far in this chapter I have attempted to summarize the existing consensus in three areas of bioethics and to suggest some instances of emerging consensus. There are also certain continuing unresolved issues and portents of new challenges for consensus in bioethics. In this section I identify a few of the ongoing issues and indicate some concerns that have not as yet received wide attention in the literature.

It may be true that hope springs eternal, but it is probably unreasonable to hope for early consensus on the vexing issue of abortion, which has been a greater and longer-lived public preoccupation in the United States than in any other country. Although new drugs such as RU-486 hold promise for fundamentally changing the conditions of the debate, it is also possible that only the locale of conflict will be changed from family planning clinics to pharmaceutical firms and even neighborhood drug stores. From the standpoint of consensus processes, the prospects for a shared point of view are undermined by wide acceptance of divergent a priori philosophical positions and institutionalized roles for advocates on either side. When people are clear about their position, and when their livelihood is wrapped up in those seemingly incompatible views, the soil for consensus is not rich, to say the very least.

The conditions are not quite identical for abortion's sibling issue, the equally ancient question of euthanasia, which has lately emerged in the form of physician-assisted suicide or, less contentiously, physician aid-in-dying. The prognosis for a working consensus on the subject is far better than in the case of abortion, if only because people are less wedded to one or another all-or-nothing viewpoint. As the population ages, and as the dying process is continually modified, further accommodations will surely be needed concerning end-of-life treatment. True respect for competently expressed wishes to abate treatment would go far to alleviate public concerns about dying tethered to machines, and the development of training programs in palliative care would greatly reduce, if not eliminate, the basis for fears about suffering at the end of life. This is not to dismiss the issue but only to indicate some elements that may provide the basis for consensus.

The converse of the physician-assisted suicide issue is that of medical futility, for here the issue is not patient control over dying but rather physician control. The futility issue is related, of course, to the limits of patient self-determination, but the status of self-determination in the pantheon of modern bioethical values is subject to challenge from quarters that are so far largely not considered in the literature. I have in mind demographic changes in American society associated with different cultural values which could in turn alter assumptions about the much-vaunted "balance" between autonomy and beneficence. For example, will the growth of Asian and Hispanic populations ultimately weaken concerns about individual self-determination and enhance familial self-determination? My own experience in a multiethnic setting has impressed me with the different expectations people bring to the doctor-patient relationship, expectations not generally captured in the bioethics literature. Will these differences persist? Or will these ethnic groups become increasingly "Americanized" and adopt the prevailing attitudes about individualism that have been embraced by earlier immigrant groups?

I have described the mini-revolution in the consensus on the participation of women of reproductive age in clinical studies. In light of those developments, new concerns will almost certainly arise about appropriate techniques for recruiting and retaining women in that age group. In the past, concerns have been expressed about coercive recruitment measures such as excessive payment. Since clinical trials typically require large numbers of subjects, and since women in this class often have responsibilities as care givers for children or older people which limit their flexibility, special measures for enrolling them, such as the provision of child care or transportation to a clinic, would be seen as unacceptably aggressive according to a "protectionist" model of research ethics. It may turn out that neither protectionism nor a radically inclusive approach, as was developed in response to AIDS, will be satisfactory as a policy concerning female subjects of reproductive age, and that a rather different model of research participation will have to be crafted.

One set of challenges in health policy that does not require lengthy discussion since it has received so much attention elsewhere is that associated with the Genome Project, the initiative to map the human genome.[25] It is worth noting the laudable effort to create a framework of moral consensus well in advance of the most far-reaching of the expected technical breakthroughs by way of the project's grant program in the ethical, legal, and social implications of this research (the ELSI program). Many of these advances may generate new threats to personal privacy, since tests will be available for genetic predispositions to certain diseases. Similarly, the reemergence of tuberculosis as an element of the HIV epidemic is a reminder that the age of highly contagious disease never really passed but only briefly abated. Following the HIV experience, however, public health policy will never be quite the same, and it is in light of that experience that future threats to public health will have to be addressed.

From the particular point of view of bioethics, no threat to whatever consensus it has managed to achieve would be as great as one that undermined its commitment to informed consent. Arthur Caplan has pointed out that the concept of informed consent to research has been articulated in a fundamentally different way from that governing informed consent for therapy, and that informed consent for therapy seems far more vulnerable to criticism. Indeed, threats to the doctrine can be anticipated from several quarters. First, the reality of illness is inherently threatening to self-determination, and the more empirical work that is done on this subject (and on the way informed consent to therapy is actually practiced), the more obvious this is likely to become. Second, demands for treatment as a matter of "right" are sure to draw continued resistance from physicians, as in the case of futile cardiopulmonary resuscitation. Third, escalating health care costs will gradually undermine the control of both patients and physicians over resources. Modifications in the doctrine of informed consent for therapy, a centerpiece of the contemporary bioethical consensus, seem inevitable.[26]

Ethics committees and the future of the bioethical consensus

I conclude this chapter with a few words on the role of ethics committees relative to the future of bioethical consensus processes in the clinical setting. Many contemporary bioethicists argue that traditional medical ethics in effect protected medical practitioners in the doctor-patient relationship from the usual constraints that liberal society imposes on human relations. That is, physicians have for generations successfully projected a paternalistic position that undercuts the liberty and equality normally expected by our liberal political philosophy. Theirs has been an ethic of duties rather than rights. These writers further claim that fundamental changes in the financing of health care are now bringing physicians under the assumptions that govern the broader society. For example, a corollary of the view that "doctor knows best" is the notion that the ethical doctor is to act only in light of his or her particular patient's needs and not those of any other party, thus also encouraging the patient's loyal subservience to his or her doctor. The growing cost of modern health care is making such a posture impossible for society to afford, these authors contend, and one result is a change in the traditional medical ethics that elegantly combined a lofty moral posture with the fee-for-service ethic.[27]

The process that these writers have described is important as we consider the implications of ethics committees. The ethics committee movement may be seen in part as a creature of the transition from the traditional medical ethics that supported an impregnable doctor-patient relationship to a new consensus about medical ethics, the implications of which are at least twofold. First, the physician must respect the liberty and equality of the patient, embodied in the doctrine of informed consent. This means that, in the process of making a knowledgeable recommendation, the doctor must recognize both the freedom of the individual to refuse unwanted interventions and her equality as a member of the polity. At the same time I assume here what has been well argued by others, that it is important to preserve the beneficence-based duties of physicians to those under their care. In the specific arena of physician-patient relations, the ethics committee movement may be understood as an attempt to promote and "troubleshoot" the new bioethical consensus that emphasizes the priority of patient self-determination while defending the continuing importance of beneficent physician behavior. The interdisciplinary membership that is usually thought to be crucial for ethics committees is thus important not only as a practical matter but also as a matter of principle, for the democratic pluralism of ethics committees itself symbolizes the democratic pluralism that conditions modern doctor-patient relations. In a departure from the past, patients are now thought of as free and equal partners in that relationship. The transformation of the physician's role has, after all, taken place over a relatively short time, and has initiated a period of uncertainty and anxiety about values which has given rise to the ethics committee.

Second, ethics committees may also play an important and highly sensitive role in any new consensus about the distribution of health care resources, especially if the view prevails that both doctors and patients have obligations to use these resources wisely. I raised this issue in the context of threats to the consensus about informed consent for therapy, but here it comes up again in a slightly different way. The patient or surrogate who wants a physician to "do everything" arguably creates an ethical problem for the physician in the modern health care marketplace, which holds out certain expectations about the way its resources will be marshaled. Previously a doctor might have been prepared to continue treatment that was physiologically useless in order to avoid conflict and provide hope. But the scarcity of certain items such as intensive care unit beds and the sheer cost of health care might in the near future generate a sense of obligation that conflicts with that strategy.

To be sure, ethics committees have largely been careful not to be, or appear to be, cost-containment devices. But cases in which "useless" therapy is a key element, particularly for incompetent patients who have not provided advance directives, are not hard to find, and will surely become more common. Cases involving competent patients or qualified surrogates who insist on continued treatment without a legitimate medical purpose will also become more common, potentially placing ethics committees in the position of suggesting limits on the positive freedom of patients to insist on expensive interventions. Forging a consensus on this issue may well be the next great ethical frontier for clinical practice beyond informed consent, and ethics committees will be key players in these developments on account of their strategic location within highly capitalized institutions. Already no lesser a figure than the editor of the *Journal of the American Medical Association* has called for ethics committees, ethics consultants, and hospital counsel to be involved in determining what counts as "futile" treatment.[28] If consensus is a goal, it requires little imagination to perceive which of these three options is most likely to enjoy wide acceptance.

Notes

1. E. F. Heely, *Medical Ethics* (Chicago: Loyola University Press, 1956), p. 45.
2. President's Commission for the Study of Ethical Problems in Medicine and Biomedical and Behavioral Research, *Deciding to Forgo Life-Sustaining Treatment: A Report on the Ethical, Medical, and Legal Issues in Treatment Decisions* (Washington, D.C.: U.S. Government Printing Office, 1983), p. 77.
3. Tom E. Beauchamp and James F. Childress, *Principles of Biomedical Ethics*, 3d ed. (New York: Oxford University Press, 1989). Although it is nearly always supposed that Beauchamp and Childress have an "application" model in mind for their principles, it is not at all clear that this is what the authors intend.
4. Albert R. Jonsen and Stephen Toulmin, *The Abuse of Casuistry* (Berkeley, Calif.: University of California Press, 1988).
5. K. Danner Clouser and Bernard Gert, "A Critique of Principlism," *Journal of Medicine and Philosophy* 15, 2 (1990): 219–36.
6. John Arras, "Getting Down to Cases: The Revival of Casuistry in Bioethics," *Journal of Medicine and Philosophy* 16, 1 (1991): 29–52.
7. Susan Sherwin, *No Longer Patient: Feminist Ethics and Health Care* (Philadelphia: Temple University Press, 1992).
8. Two bioethicists have argued that courts have shown a distinctly paternalistic pattern in dealing with "right-to-die" cases involving female patients. See Stephen H. Miles and Allison August, "Courts, Gender, and 'the Right to Die,'" *Law, Medicine, and Health Care* 18, 1, 2 (1990): 85–95.
9. Alan Meisel, "The Legal Consensus about Forgoing Life-Sustaining Treatment: Its Status and Prospects," *Kennedy Institute of Ethics Journal* 2, 4 (1992): 315.
10. H. Tristram Engelhardt, Jr., *The Foundations of Bioethics* (New York: Oxford University Press, 1986).
11. *Grace Plaza of Great Neck, Inc. v. Murray Elbaum* 162 N.Y.S. 3265. In 1993 the highest court in New York State ruled that the nursing home was entitled to payment

because it acted in good faith in seeking legal clarification of the family's rights to decline treatment. In the meantime, it was obligated to continue treatment.

12. Nancy Rhoden, "Litigating Life and Death," *Harvard Law Review* 102, 2 (1988): 375–446.

13. Jan Hare, Clara Platt, and Carrie Nelson, "Agreement Between Patients and Their Self-Selected Surrogates on Difficult Medical Decisions," *Archives of Internal Medicine* 152, 5 (1992): 1049–54.

14. Robert Weir, *Abating Treatment with Critically Ill Patients* (New York: Oxford University Press, 1990).

15. Ellen Fox and Carol Stocking, "Ethics Consultants' Recommendations for Life-Prolonging Treatment of Patients in a Persistent Vegetative State," *New England Journal of Medicine* 270, 21 (1993): 2578–82.

16. Ibid., p. 2581.

17. Paul Ramsey, *The Patient as Person* (New Haven: Yale University Press, 1970).

18. Robert Levine, *Ethics and the Regulation of Clinical Research*, 2d ed. (Baltimore: Urban and Schwarzenberg, 1986).

19. Ibid., pp. 8–9.

20. For background material on this issue, see Anna C. Mastroianni, Ruth Faden, and Daniel Federman, eds., *Women and Health Research: Ethical and Legal Issues of Including Women in Clinical Studies*, vol. 1 and 2 (Washington, D.C.: National Academy Press, 1994).

21. Jonathan D. Moreno and Howard Minkoff, "HIV Infection During Pregnancy," *Clinical Obstetrics and Gynecology* 35, 4 (1992): 813–20; and Howard Minkoff, Jonathan D. Moreno, and Kathleen E. Powderly, "Fetal Protection and Women's Access to Clinical Trials," *Journal of Women's Health* 1, 2 (1992): 37–41.

22. Ronald Bayer, *Private Acts, Social Consequences* (New York: Free Press, 1989).

23. Gail Povar and Jonathan D. Moreno, "Hippocrates and the HMO," *Annals of Internal Medicine* 109, 5 (1988): 419–24.

24. E. Haavi Morreim, *Balancing Act: The New Medical Ethics of Medicine's New Economics* (Dordrecht: Kluwer Academic Publishers, 1991).

25. Thomas H. Murray, "The Genome Project and Genetic Testing: Ethical Implications," in *The Genome, Ethics and the Law: Issues in Genetic Testing* (Washington, D.C.: American Association for the Advancement of Science, 1992), pp. 49–78.

26. Arthur L. Caplan, "Can Informed Consent be Saved?," Division of Humanities in Medicine Fifth Anniversary Colloquium, April 29, 1993. SUNY Health Science Center at Brooklyn, New York. Stephen Wear has gone further than any other writer to date in attempting to specify different levels of informed consent depending on the circumstances and the patient's wishes. See Stephen Wear, *Informed Consent: Patient Autonomy and Physician Beneficence Within Clinical Medicine* (Dordrecht: Kluwer Academic Publishers, 1993).

27. Troyen Brennen, *Just Doctoring: Medical Ethics in the Liberal State* (Berkeley: University of California Press, 1993); see also Morreim, *Balancing Act*.

28. George Lundberg, "American Health Care System Management Objectives: The Aura of Inevitability Becomes Incarnate," editorial, *JAMA* 269, 19 (1993): 2554–55.

3

Analyzing Consensus

Of Philoctetes and Proteus

In a provocative image Bruce Jennings has compared the role of consensus in moral philosophy to that of Philoctetes in Greek mythology: "Cursed by the gods, he carried an open wound that would not heal and was thus loathsome to men; but without the bow he carried, right could not prevail."[1] Consensus is an inescapable feature of moral decision making in social life, but one that causes anxiety among ethical theorists. As Jennings notes, it reinforces patterns of power, channels and neutralizes conflict, and diffuses responsibility, thereby supporting established patterns of domination.[2] Yet appeals for and to consensus are ubiquitous. And without consensus how could any view, including that which is right, prevail in human affairs except by coercion? Moreover, whatever its failings, consensus at least suggests the possibility that particularistic self-concern may be transformed into a sense of what persons value in common. Can we effect a reconciliation with Philoctetes?

Greek mythology provides another pointed image for this study. Proteus, a sea god, was capable of assuming many different forms. A large part of the social utility of consensus resides in its protean nature, for mention of the word can smooth all sorts of situations that seem pregnant with conflict. Its ambiguity allows the parties an assent accompanied sometimes by a vague sense of relief. Paradoxically, in order to reconcile with Philoctetes, a task that entails clarifying the moral status of consensus, we put Proteus at hazard.

In this chapter I explore three philosophical distinctions that can be applied to the concept of consensus: descriptive and prescriptive consensus, substantive and procedural consensus, and consensus as process and as product. These distinctions are finally less useful than might be thought. In each case analysis casts doubt on the practical differences among them. Nonetheless, I stress the practical importance of distinguishing between consensus and compromise. The main idea here is that the epistemology and ethics of consensus on the one hand and the sociology of consensus on the other have more to do with each other than we are accustomed to thinking. Although his domain may be somewhat diminished by the ascent of Philoctetes, at the end of the day Proteus still stands.

Not only is the idea of consensus amorphous and ethically suspect, but also it is exceedingly complex, subject to analysis from sociological, political, and philosophical perspectives. Before we proceed to the philosophical distinctions, let us identify the social scientific perspectives for later use. The sociological standpoint mainly involves describing the various ways consensus can be used to encourage a sense of social cohesion. Thus, from a functional point of view, a social system may require more or less explicit general agreement, depending on the circumstances. When the stakes are high, social control mechanisms such as norms and values may ensure cohesion, at least up to a point. As I elaborate in chapter 7, consensus itself plays an important role in social control. (A terminological aside: I take expressions such as "general agreement" and "collective opinion" to be synonymous with consensus, but general agreement can include consensus by acquiescence as well as more active forms of consensus development. This point is obvious to sociologists but not to philosophers, who often think of consensus in connection with an idealized model of social contractors.)

In those cases where a question is regarded as trivial, a group signals this by acquiescing to the status quo or to direction given by authority figures. At the other extreme, potentially controversial questions may also be decided by acquiescence if a group gives a sufficiently high value to the preservation of cohesion. Matters that are either not likely to engender social conflict or are regarded as too important to be left to mere passive agreement could be submitted to a "head count," referred to in parliamentary terms as "the sense of the house," so that members can be sure that a rough majority of their fellows concur. Explicit voting can sometimes reveal a consensus, though most often it is avoided if that would jeopardize social tranquillity.[3] A population may also be acquiescent, however, when it is under duress, a state of affairs that could not without distortion be characterized as consensus. I present these and other sociological and social psychological considerations in chapters 7 and 8.

The political standpoint is mainly concerned with the several functional forms of consensus in authorizing government action. Thus, in *permissive consensus* the public is prepared for policies so the government will later be able to pursue them. Expert panels are frequently convened by government bodies to help prepare the public for some new idea or program. *Supportive consensus* refers to a practice by competing groups within a government (e.g., rival political parties) to continue some settled policy regardless of which group is currently in power. Note that this form of consensus may have little or nothing to do with democratic processes, for it refers to cooperation among established rival powers rather than to consent of the governed. In *decisive consensus* the polity authorizes the government to take some particular step, though again the government may not be one that on the whole operates through consent. An example would be a people's decision to authorize a despot's defense of the homeland from a rapacious foreign invader.[4] These categories are drawn from political science, not political philosophy. The basis in political philosophy for an authorized moral consensus in a liberal, democratic, and diverse society is my concern in chapter 4.

Procedural and substantive consensus

A relatively familiar philosophical distinction is that between procedural consensus and substantive consensus. According to the standard account, *procedural consensus* is operative when there is agreement about the rules or methods that will be followed in resolving actual or possible conflicts about substantive matters. In turn, *substantive consensus* is agreement with one of a number of alternative and conflicting points of view. There is logical "slack" running in both directions between procedural and substantive consensus; from the fact that there is one sort of consensus the other may not be inferred.

The concept of a procedural consensus is valuable in that it highlights the fact that consensus is never just a static end (though it is usually described as such in ordinary discourse) but is also an element that characterizes the whole deliberative process. Peter Caws further distinguishes three different "moments in the process": "the initial situation of the participants" (which he calls procedural consensus), "the ways in which they change their positions, and the collective judgment that emerges (if it does)."[5] This point alone would be enough to establish that some sort and degree of consensus is a necessary feature of the entire process. But Isaac Levi goes further, stating that "a background of shared agreement" of a *substantive* nature must be present at the outset if there is to be any hope of an ultimate agreement.[6]

An example of a minimal background of shared agreement can be found in Engelhardt's bioethical theory, in which he posits mutual respect among the parties to a controversy and the concomitant agreement to forgo the use of force as essential to the peaceable resolution of moral controversy.[7] Liberal political philosophies in general posit the abstract value of personal autonomy, from which more "contentful" values, both procedural and substantive, follow. By contentful I mean values that are relatively more specific, more highly articulated in their meanings, than others. At the other extreme, in actual instances of moral controversy such as might be encountered in a clinical ethics conference, the parties already share a rich array of beliefs, ranging from factual medical information to moral values. This sort of scenario exemplifies a highly ramified background consensus, one with widely recognized implications, including agreement on matters of substance as well as procedure, without which management of real-world differences would be but a fantasy. It can be shown that even in Engelhardt's "foundational" scenario which proceeds from the abstract and general value of personal autonomy, substantive consensus cannot wholly be avoided. For the parties to a controversy must be prepared to tolerate one another, and in order to do that they must find one another tolerable. That this is a nontrivial factor is illustrated by the fact that a wider "community of tolerance" may be achievable, to use Allan Gibbard's phrase, but not desirable. Consider, for example, a community of tolerance with neo-Nazis. Depending on one's particular beliefs, it could be argued that not everyone is due respect.[8]

At any rate, this analysis suggests that there is less to the distinction between substantive values and procedural consensus than meets the eye. Of far more importance are the questions *how much* and *what kind of* content a value has. Not only are substantive values hard to avoid, even in the most abstract setting, but also, depending on the circumstances, procedural standards can have substantive implications. Consider, for example, a parliamentary body that is divided about what rule to adopt concerning the majority needed to overturn an executive veto. Is a simple majority not enough, implying a weak executive? Is three quarters too much, implying an excessively powerful legislature? The procedural options entail substantive constitutional issues.

In his recent work John Rawls has invoked the idea of "overlapping consensus," a spatial metaphor intended to suggest that the members of a pluralistic society will agree on some ideas and values but will not all agree on the same ones. To Rawls this suggests that it is often prudent to refrain from attempts to gain social agreement on certain intractable controversies.[9] Here again it is the details of the values that are important rather than whether they are procedural or substantive. Furthermore, in comparison with the rather limited reach of the procedural-substantive distinction, the idea that consensus involves overlap or "breadth" is intriguing; it will return as an important idea in chapter 4. It also leads one to wonder about consensus in terms of "depth."

A useful example of deep consensus is Stephen Toulmin's report of his experiences as a consultant for the National Commission for the Protection of Human Subjects of Biomedical and Behavioral Research. Toulmin claims that the commissioners had far less difficulty reaching agreement on specific policies than was the case when each attempted to identify his or her own moral reasoning behind the common conclusion.[10] Now we are in a position to see the overlap in its horizontal as well as its vertical dimensions. That is, the roughly overlapping beliefs that imperfectly hold the members of a pluralistic society together could be "shallow," in the sense that there is general agreement about particular cases, or "deep," in the sense that there is general agreement about principles. These possibilities are currently being discussed by authors working on methodological problems in bioethics as the debate between casuists and deductivists.[11]

Descriptive and prescriptive consensus

Again according to a familiar distinction, ethics may be descriptive, as in a sociological account of the moral views of a particular group, or prescriptive, as in a philosophical or theological text that commends a particular point of view on a moral question. In either case it is always sensible to ask whether there is merit in the view that is held by a large number of people (descriptive ethics) or that is defended by argument or appeal to authority (prescriptive ethics). Consensus ethics is usually thought to be a variation of descriptive ethics, as it reports the more or less settled and predominant views of some population. In the discussion that follows I use the terms *view*, *belief*, and *perspective* interchangeably, with the further understanding that a belief may be accurately ascribed to a person when that person is willing to act on that belief.

Now, a descriptive ethical account may itself yield a consensus that is either descriptive or prescriptive. *Descriptive consensus* refers to a widespread opinion that something is the case, while *prescriptive consensus* refers to a widespread opinion that commends that belief to others. It may seem strange to distinguish between what people say are their moral beliefs and what people say are moral beliefs that they would commend to others, since surely (on pain of inconsistency) if I have a certain belief I would commend it to all others who are similarly situated. But I am not certain that this is always the case, logic to the contrary notwithstanding. For example, a public opinion survey might well find a *descriptive* pro-life consensus, while a survey of the same population could find a *prescriptive* pro-choice consensus (i.e., "I would not have an abortion, but I would not impose this view on others").

In practice, descriptive and prescriptive consensus can easily be conflated, giving a descriptive consensus of expert opinion a moral status it does not necessarily deserve. For example, an international survey of professionals in the field of genetics inquired about the morality of selective abortion on grounds of fetal sex, among other questions.[12] The results *described* the professionals' views on that issue, but it is not clear that the professionals surveyed would also *prescribe* these views to others, especially those who feel constrained not to recommend their views to colleagues from different cultures. In other words, the questions took the logical form "Would you . . . ?" rather than "Should one . . . ?"

Although it is not at all clear that the genetics professionals' expertise gives them any special qualifications that would commend their ethical consensus to anyone else, it is a safe bet that many lay people will receive their views as prescriptively authoritative, especially in regard to ethics in genetics. The descriptive-prescriptive distinction reminds us not to take expert views at face value, and there is an unassailable wisdom about this. Yet in practice it seems odd not to accord expertise a measure of deference. After all, one important reason why we identify individuals as experts is precisely to obviate the need to investigate certain questions ourselves. Again, one comes away with the sense that the descriptive-prescriptive distinction is important but practically limited.

Consensus as process and as product

A ready philosophical criticism of my project in this book is that it errs in its preoccupation with the *process* of ethical decision making rather than with what "really" counts, its *product*. To put this criticism in terms that were not so long ago part of the bread and butter of the philosophy of science, worries about the moral authority of consensus processes rather than intellectual argument confuse the "context of discovery" with the "context of justification." On this view, people may reach a state of moral belief in all kinds of ways, from poetic reverie to positive reinforcement (the process of discovery), but all that matters is the extent to which the ideas themselves are legitimate (justifying the product).

The process-product distinction is no longer taken to be decisive in contemporary philosophy, nor is it generally held that the two contexts can be so neatly differentiated. At least in the realm of actual social practices, and particularly in the development of what is sometimes called social ethics, it is patent that the admission of intellectual arguments as sound is itself an unavoidably social process. This is not to deny the role of expertise or justification but only to acknowledge the setting in which these elements must come into play. Moreover, the process by which a belief is attained is commonly used in defense of the product, the belief itself. Thus, in defending a result of moral deliberation we may call attention to the "unbiased" nature of the procedure, one in which all relevant factors have been fairly and properly taken into account; in jurisprudence this is known as due process. Conversely, if the process has been corrupted or distorted, this is widely taken as a prima facie reason to think that the result of that process is likely to be erroneous in some way.

Recent theoretical discussions in bioethics illustrate this point. As I noted in the previous chapter, bioethical theorists commonly referred to as principlists have identified certain moral principles (usually autonomy, beneficence, nonmaleficence, and justice) for the guidance they can provide us in dealing with particular problems or cases.[13] These principles are essential elements of what has become the dominant methodology in bioethics. Casuists have criticized principlism on the ground that moral problems cannot be treated by appeal to abstract principles, nor can cases be handled independently of other cases; rather, they can be dealt with only by comparing and contrasting the elements of specific cases and assembling a set of guiding maxims from particular judgments.[14] Casuistry, along with other insurgent movements in bioethical theory such as feminism[15] and the care perspective,[16] has reintroduced a concern for the process of moral deliberation as bound up with its product.

In their most recent explication of their views, Tom Beauchamp and James Childress argue that their approach is amenable to the casuists' concerns. In fact, these principlists themselves embrace the salient point that formalistic differentiation between the process of moral deliberation and the justification of the results of moral deliberation is untenable.[17] This conclusion has implications beyond consensus theory itself, as it is also suggestive for a consensus-oriented view of bioethics. Such an account would frame the institution of bioethics in terms of social as well as philosophical considerations. In the last several chapters I elaborate on some elements of such a standpoint.

Consensus and compromise

Although I have depreciated the practical differences represented in three distinctions relevant to consensus, the one I introduce now is quite important. Consensus and compromise are ideas that we have no trouble using differently in ordinary language, but they are not so easy to distinguish when we are challenged to do so. One source of confusion is the fact that consensus involves reaching agreement on one of a number of theoretically available compromises. This is the typical situation in a negotiation between parties with differing interests. Each party enters the scene with a more or less fixed agenda. The strategy is to find an accommodation that preserves the nonnegotiable values of the respective parties to the controversy.[18]

But the model of negotiation should not casually be applied to a situation in which there is general and genuine uncertainty about the best course of action, for this is one in which consensus rather than compromise is the operative concept. Compromise, again, suggests that parties to a controversy have entered the scene with more or less fixed preferences. Consensus carries no such baggage; it suggests an openness to unanticipated possibilities and points of view. At a deeper level, it holds out the prospect that individuals will themselves change as a result of the process, that they will achieve perspectives that had not been available to them before. By contrast, compromise implies at most a deeper appreciation of one's preexistent concerns, including which ones are held most dear.

Furthermore, in a negotiated compromise model both parties enter the bargaining room having a fairly good idea what their basic interests are, with the intention at least to defend if not advance them. Whatever compromise is to be reached will be constrained by those a priori positions. Consensus, however, implies no such clarity about one's particular interests, nor even necessarily which interests are at stake in the current deliberations. The identification of relevant concerns as well as their respective priority may itself be part of the consensus process. Thus, in reaching a consensus about one potential settlement or another, the participants might discover features about their preferences that emerge as they consider the various theoretically acceptable alternatives, features that did not occur to them prior to entertaining the possible compromises.

Seen in this light, some bioethical controversies can be readily identified as situations in which consensus is far less likely than compromise. Abortion is easily the best example of an issue about which consensus seems beyond our grasp and the best we can do is achieve a stable compromise. Again, this is because the parties have entered the situation with fixed views that are amenable to modification only at the margins. This is what is meant when it is said that an ethical issue has become "politicized," since individuals are wedded to their positions, and the amelioration of social paralysis will have to take those positions as the de facto starting points. Yet, many bioethical issues, while they certainly contain political elements, have not been captured by those elements in the public debate. The other ancient ethical issue of euthanasia is an example of one in which hard and fast public positions have not as yet eliminated the possibility of a new consensus on physician-assisted suicide. To the extent, however, that any other bioethical issue becomes pulled into the maelstrom of abortion, at least in American society, the possibility of consensus is surely threatened.

Unlike the distinctions between consensus as substantive and procedural, as descriptive and prescriptive, and as process and product, that between consensus and compromise is critical in social practice. Without being clear about what kind of situation one is in, one cannot know what sort of resolution is practically possible. Usually a situation in which the realistic goal is compromise offers at best the prospect of a modus vivendi, an arrangement that makes living feasible in spite of continuing difficulties, whereas a situation in which one may reasonably aspire to consensus can, for well or ill, involve a true social transformation.

My proposed reform in the use of compromise and consensus has implications for bioethical commentary. For example, in his carefully developed and qualified vision of communitarian health care, Ezekiel Emanuel ventures a usage of the word consensus that I would qualify. When two parties share a basic commitment but disagree about each other's view or interpretation, then the resolution of that disagreement is not what I would call a consensus, but a compromise based on the underlying consensus.[19] Emanuel also identifies consensus too closely with straightforward voting procedures.[20] If my analysis has merit, then there is need for a clearer understanding of consensus processes and of information from the social sciences in assessing moral consensus in a liberal and pluralistic society.

Metaphysics and moral consensus

We must now begin to face the vexed philosophical question of what a moral consensus is "about," of what to make of the status of statements about morality, including those that are accepted by consensus. Certain extreme views reveal confused and even dangerous assumptions that can be held about consensus in bioethics but that can be corrected by a more carefully considered account of moral consensus. These two views, which I will call bioethical platonism and bioethical relativism, must be dispatched early on.

Bioethical platonism (the lower-case *p* is used so as not to overidentify this view with a particular historical figure) is really an insistence on a transcendental foundation, a timeless and immutable moral Good. Without such a foundation, it may be thought, any one bioethical consensus is as good as any other. But a bioethics without transcendental foundations need not be a bioethics without principles, guidelines, maxims, or canons. Its "grounding" can be of this world rather than of some ideal world that is alleged to be immanent in this one, with reference to data from the social sciences and the material of human experience rather than intuitive idealism. When I articulate my naturalistic theory of consensus in bioethics, I appeal, for example, to moral psychology and the pattern of human inquiry.

As serious a threat to an understanding of consensus in bioethics as platonism is relativism. The implications, or even the precise meaning, of moral relativism are sources of long-standing debate in moral philosophy, and I have nothing original to add. In a book about consensus in bioethics, however, it would be irresponsible not to acknowledge that the historic emergence of the field is closely associated with the horrific abuses of concentration camp inmates during the Holocaust, and with the scandalous treatment of vulnerable subject populations in Tuskegee and at Willowbrook. Surely many regard those experiences as powerful warnings about the hazards of "doing ethics without a net," which could lead to a "might makes right" attitude of the crudest sort.

It is important to distinguish between relativism in the minds of those responsible for these acts and relativism as a philosophical attitude toward the morality they exemplify. The Nazis, for instance, were not moral relativists; quite the contrary. Nazism and other forms of fascism maintain passionate and ironclad commitments to absolutist doctrines of race, clan, and soil that do not admit even the possibility of countervailing evidence. Indeed, Hitler and other fascist theorists regarded Western democracy as hopelessly corrupted by "relativistic" attitudes which they sought to replace. Intellectuals of Jewish background, for example, were suspect precisely because they were thought to be "rootless cosmopolitans" who as a group did not identify with a single moral standard that transcended any particular set of cultural values.

These reflections are helpful reminders that deference to an alleged moral reality antecedent to and independent of human experience is as much a threat to humanity as moral relativism. Yet relativism remains a danger in a somewhat different way, in the form of reluctance to criticize the Nazi "moral consensus." As many authors have pointed out, liberalism and tolerance should not be permitted to degenerate into an "anything goes" attitude. Bioethics must take care not to cede claim to moral authority in a culture that tends toward cynicism and skepticism. A common disconcerting experience of contemporary teachers of the humanities and social sciences is a reluctance among students to criticize heinous acts committed in other times and places, a reluctance founded on a distorted notion of tolerance.

More promising as a source of guidance on the philosophy of moral consensus are the results of an intensive discussion among Anglo-American moral philosophers about the status of moral claims. Following Geoffrey Sayre-McCord, three positions can be distinguished: *subjectivism*, according to which the truth conditions of a moral claim (what makes a moral claim true) make essential reference to an individual; *intersubjectivism* if they make essential reference to group conventions; and *objectivism* if they make no essential reference to people or their conventions.[21] Although moral consensus seems to be a form of intersubjectivism, it could as easily be analyzed in reference to the separate beliefs of all the individuals who participate in the consensus, or in terms of an objective state of affairs to which all the identical beliefs of the participants refer (the "Moral Reality"). Which of these three positions one holds turns out to make very little difference to particular moral claims, whether arrived at by consensus or by some other means. The difference lies in what philosophical sense one makes of what a moral consensus refers to, and unless one is interested in moral epistemology, that is not enough of a difference to worry about.

With one significant exception: for a certain distinguished and influential version of objectivism, even a moral consensus that referred to or "agreed with" an independent Moral Reality could not represent the truth but would merely be a "right opinion." I have observed that Socrates (or at least Plato's Socrates, the paradigmatic objectivist) did not seem to think that a consensus could be true for the right reasons, as though there were something about consensus processes that necessarily contaminated a search for knowledge. That is, not only is democracy not guided by a knowledge of the Good, but activities associated with group deliberation are at best irrelevant to coming to know the Good. The philosopher-kings will of course all agree about the Good, but not because they have discussed it with one another. (On this view, the vaunted dialogue form is a pedagogic model rather than a philosophic technique; it would seem that the logos speaks only to those who already know what it says.) Thus, what philosophers call justified true belief always falls short of knowledge, according to this tradition. It appears that Plato's Socrates held this view, not only as a result of his metaphysics of ideal Forms but also in connection with his critical perspective on democratic processes. No doubt the trial and execution of the historical Socrates did nothing to disabuse Plato of his skepticism about the deliberative potential of the crowd. This jaundiced view of the possibilities for consensus is deeply rooted in our Western philosophical traditions and presents a persistent intellectual challenge to a constructive account of moral consensus.

Equally rooted in Western philosophy is the suspicion that moral truth is, both in principle and in fact, less likely to be achieved by groups, which are vulnerable to the corruptions of political processes and interpersonal dynamics, than by well-informed and reflective individuals. This view, a version of objectivism, may well be associated with a desiccated mythology of the heroic individual in a lonely quest for Truth, but, however discredited, it continues to exercise a strong grip on the minds of many. A modern version holds any consensus-based conclusion about ethics to be an instance of the naturalistic fallacy, or the allegedly inappropriate inference of statements of value from statements of fact. An example would be inferring "This patient ought to be sterilized" (a value statement) from "This duly authorized committee finds that this patient ought to be sterilized" (a fact statement).

As with the three distinctions I assessed earlier, it seems hard to deny the logic of the fact-value distinction. Yet again I believe that this is often a case of a distinction without a difference. The fact that we hold a certain moral value is an instance of two intellectually distinguishable elements (the fact and the value), but in the realm of human affairs we cannot differentiate the fact from the value. A familiar example of this difficulty is the moral status of the fertilized ovum, which some believe can be described in biological terms without reference to any moral character it may be alleged to have as a potential person, while others believe that this would be an essentially incomplete description.

Not only does ordinary life frequently present us with situations in which facts and values are hard to disentangle, but also it is hard to see how human institutions (at least those in states claiming to be liberal democracies) could practically function without routinely relying on consensus about matters that include a mixture of facts and values. This routine reliance on consensus can be said to persist on a first-order level and a second-order level. The machinery of organized social life in all its dealings surely requires the lubricant of common agreement. Furthermore, in a second-order sense there is also a social and psychological need to see that collective opinion as by and large the right opinion. The analysis of the legitimation processes of consensus views is normally the province of sociology, which concerns itself, for example, with the formal and informal processes through which bodies such as ethics commissions or ethics committees gain or lose their perceived legitimacy in the polity or the institution. The sociological perspective emphasizes the social and political realities of consensus decision making and does not trouble itself with the traditional philosophical critique of consensus. However superficial this approach may seem to those who are mainly interested in normative problems, the sociological view makes available analytic methods that are enlightening with respect to the moral authority of consensus processes. Some of these methods are reviewed and applied in later chapters.

I do not pretend to have vanquished with these remarks the fact-value distinction, nor is that my goal. In any case it would be arrogant to think that it could

be so easily done, for the literature on this subject is immense and sophisticated. Rather, my aim is to criticize a simplistic conception of the relation between
facts and values. If progress is to be made in improving our understanding of
bioethics in the light of actual social practices, then it is more useful to regard
facts and values as moments in iterated consensus processes. Consider again
the proposition that the moment of conception is due respect as the beginning
of human life. The insistence that this proposition must express either a fact or
a value is not terribly helpful, since that is exactly what the abortion debate is
about.

Levels of consensus

I want to return now to the idea of deep consensus, which was characterized earlier as relevant to agreement about principles and not only cases. This section and
the one that follows anticipate two later chapters on ethics panels. When commissions or committees address cases or policies that engage ethical problems properly so called, they rely on consensus partly because of the unsettled nature of the
issues. That issues are unsettled imposes two related challenges on the panelists:
the political challenge of finding a nontrivial formulation that will bring as many
as possible under its rubric and the philosophical challenge of dealing with genuine uncertainty in an intellectually responsible and morally justifiable way. These
issues may involve either ethical ambiguity or ethical conflict. The former occurs
when some interpretation of the underlying relevant ethical principles is required,
for there is lack of clarity about the proper interpretation of the principles for the
present case or for the policy being proposed, but there is no apparent disagreement about the rightness of the principles themselves. This sort of dilemma involves disagreement about the rightness of the way the principles have been
brought to bear on this case or proposed policy, or in other words the interpretation of the principles. Thus, in one instance what is required of the panel is consensus about application of principles, while in the second instance what is required is consensus about principles, or deep consensus.

   If this account of two levels of consensus is sound, then it appears that agreement at one level does not guarantee agreement at the other. Ethics committee
deliberation may not go so deep as the discussion of the merit of principles themselves. If Toulmin's account of the National Commission can be generalized (an
account which is controversial, as we will see in chapter 5), that suggests that striving for agreement at the level of deep consensus is quite exceptional. Rather, according to Toulmin, what seems more routine is the effort to reach consensus at
the level of cases simpliciter. Reactions and intuitions are exchanged by committee members following a review of medical, psychosocial, and legal factors. Rarely
are underlying values questioned, except perhaps by a philosopher or theologian
who happens to be a committee member. Thus, in reference to his experience as

a consultant to and staff member of the National Commission, Toulmin reports that discussions about principles themselves were infrequent. More divisive were views about how to apply particular principles or what principles should be used to reach a conclusion about which there was agreement. The differences among the commissioners did not reveal themselves until each gave "reasons" for his or her conclusion. Toulmin explains this phenomenon by appeal to the nature of the deliberations on the "hard cases" up for review: "[The members] inquired what particular conflicts of claim or interest were exemplified in them, and they usually ended by balancing off those claims in very similar ways."[22]

Toulmin's account may resonate for those who have participated in similar deliberations. One may find oneself in a group that reaches more or less the same conclusion for different reasons. It seems those differences can be the result of interpreting or weighing the same principles somewhat differently; or they may arise from selecting entirely different principles that happen in this instance to lead to the same conclusion. From this Toulmin draws the conclusion that attention to cases allows the degree of certitude appropriate to practical reasoning in ethics, that is, a level of confidence in one's conclusions that can be reasonably expected in a nondeductive area of inquiry.

If Toulmin is right about this, a particular worry arises: does it follow that the members of an ethics commission or committee might be better off not to examine too closely their reasons for taking one view or another lest they discover the depth of their differences and compromise their ability to function together? Then how can the panel be sure that its decisions are well founded if the results of group self-consciousness about principled differences are so threatening that self-study is avoided? This conundrum does not necessarily represent either the defeat of the idea of an ethics panel or an escape from moral or intellectual responsibility on the part of its members. It does suggest that closer attention must be paid to the social realities of moral deliberation in small groups.

The more one considers these complex questions, the more one is struck that the challenge of finding consensus on basic values, which is often taken to be the most serious problem of moral consensus, is actually eclipsed by problems much closer to the ground. Indeed, it seems likely that straightforward conflicts of basic values are rare, so broad and bland are those values. Thus, we may agree in general that "respect for life" is a basic ethical principle yet discover that we interpret it or balance it against other values quite differently. Some philosophers would say that in that case we do not really hold the same idea at all. How, then, can the members be sure that they have truly reached the "same" conclusion rather than a superficial and finely crafted linguistic compromise that will collapse at the first sign of a hard case? Leaving the epistemological problem aside, we see clearly that even when a number of people believe that the idea to which they assent is the same, there is no guarantee that action will be uniform. Again, it appears that attention to the nature of deliberation itself is important.

Affirming consensus

Finally, there is a philosophically interesting empirical feature of consensus that is familiar to experienced members of consensus-oriented groups but the significance of which appears to have escaped notice. Often it seems that the group's determination that there be a consensus on a particular matter is highlighted in a specific moment of the process. Thus, at a certain point the chair often utters a consensus-affirming statement such as, "Well, I suppose we have a consensus," theoretically giving all members the opportunity to respond along a spectrum ranging from active assent to acquiescence to active dissent. Interestingly, even if there is dissent from the majority view, the group may still decide that there is a consensus; even those who do not agree with the majority view might agree that there is a consensus, however grudgingly. They may do this for many reasons, including (as I have already mentioned) the future amity of the group. This is a remarkable feature of group consensus, for no such possibility is open when the process requires a vote. Those who dissent cannot simply agree that there is unanimity when there is none, unless they change their vote. But the idea of consensus is so ambiguous (involving notions such as the relation between the idea of consensus and that of unanimity) that it is useful in preserving a level of group cohesion in spite of disagreements on specific points.

A philosophically interesting aspect of this phenomenon is that the chair's consensus-affirming statement, "Well, I suppose we have a consensus," has what might be called a *semiperformative* character. Performative utterances are speech acts that, uttered by the right person under the right circumstances, also accomplish certain functions. Declarations by authorities are the most obvious example. Thus, the act of stating, "I now pronounce you husband and wife," when uttered by the right person under the right circumstances, creates a new state of affairs.[23] The word calls into being, as it were.

I call affirmations of consensus *semi*performative utterances because, unlike full-blown performatives, they do not usually create a new state of affairs so much as certify it for public recognition, unless, that is, the committee chair is attempting to impose his or her will on the process before agreement has actually been reached, in which case the affirmation may indeed be performative. More usually consensus affirmations are akin to the jury foreman's stating the findings of the jury in open court. The findings have already been made, but the foreman's announcement does more than simply punctuate the process, for it is an essential ritual. In comparison to the formal ritual of the courtroom, the committee chair's declaration is part of an informal but also terribly important ritual. The consensus affirmation is a sort of social gestalt mechanism, for without it there would not be a shared sense of completion. It seems, therefore, to be a critical part of the informal consensus process.

With this last subject we see how understanding the actual workings of consensus can illuminate social decision making. Thus, in much of this book I attempt to ground ethics panels in actual social practices, including studies of their history, legal role, political status, and internal social structure. My aim in these discussions is to create an empirical background for a philosophical appraisal of moral deliberation in small groups. That task will be taken up after the discussion of consensus and political liberalism in the next chapter. For the time being I hope that I have conveyed in this chapter the degree to which careful thinking about consensus involves challenging familiar distinctions and reveals it to be a tightly woven fabric of epistemic, ethical, and sociological threads.

Notes

1. Bruce Jennings, "Possibilities of Consensus: Toward Democratic Moral Discourse," *Journal of Medicine and Philosophy* 16, 4 (1991): 447.
2. Ibid., p. 452.
3. Manfred Stanley, *The Technological Conscience: Survival and Dignity in an Age of Expertise* (New York: Free Press, 1991).
4. Key, *Public Opinion and American Democracy.*
5. Peter Caws, "Committees and Consensus: How Many Heads Are Better Than One?," *Journal of Medicine and Philosophy* 16, 4 (1991): 375–91.
6. Isaac Levi, "Consensus as Shared Agreement and Outcome of Inquiry," *Synthèse* 62, 1 (1985): 3–11.
7. Engelhardt, *Foundations of Bioethics.*
8. Allan Gibbard, *Wise Choices, Apt Feelings: A Theory of Normative Judgment* (Cambridge, Mass.: Harvard University Press, 1990).
9. John Rawls, "Kantian Constructivism in Moral Theory: The Dewey Lectures 1980," *Journal of Philosophy* 77, 9 (1980): 515–72.
10. Stephen Toulmin, "How Medicine Saved the Life of Ethics," in *New Directions in Ethics*, ed. J. P. DeMarco and R. M. Fox (New York: Routledge and Kegan Paul, 1986), pp. 265–81.
11. Andrew Lustig, "Perseverations on a Critical Theme," *Journal of Medicine and Philosophy* 18, 5 (1993): 491–502.
12. Dorothy C. Wertz, "Lessons from an International Survey of Medical Geneticists," in *Ethical Issues of Molecular Genetics in Psychiatry*, ed. R. J. Sram, V. Bulyzhenkov, L. Prilipko, and Y. Christen (New York: Springer-Verlag, 1991), pp. xxx.
13. Tom E. Beauchamp and James F. Childress, *Principles of Biomedical Ethics*, 4th ed. (New York: Oxford University Press, 1994).
14. Jonsen and Toulmin, *Abuse of Casuistry.*
15. Sherwin, *No Longer Patient.*
16. Warren T. Reich, "Speaking of Suffering: A Moral Account of Compassion," *Soundings* 72, 1 (1989): 83–108.
17. Beauchamp and Childress, *Principles of Biomedical Ethics*, 4th ed., pp. 92–99.
18. For the most complete account of compromise in bioethics, see Martin Benjamin, *Splitting the Difference: Compromise and Integrity in Ethics and Politics* (Lawrence: University Press of Kansas, 1990).

19. Emanuel, *Ends of Human Life*, pp. 168–69.
20. Ibid., p. 182.
21. Geoffrey Sayre-McCord, "Introduction: The Many Moral Realisms," in *Essays on Moral Realism*, ed. Geoffrey Sayre-McCord (Ithaca, N.Y.: Cornell University Press, 1991), pp. 1–23.
22. Toulmin, "How Medicine Saved the Life of Ethics," pp. 270–71.
23. J. L. Austin, *How To Do Things with Words* (Oxford: Oxford University Press, 1962).

4

Liberalism and the Moral Authority of Consensus

Consensus and liberalism

The previous chapter was mainly concerned with the epistemological and ethical issues involved in the idea of moral consensus. Chapter 2 reviewed some of the main elements of the contemporary bioethical consensus. In this chapter I describe the political rationale for the authority of moral consensus within the framework of our society's liberal philosophy and surface some of the problems that the idea of moral consensus poses for that widely held framework. I also suggest some solutions to these problems, arguing that in a liberal and pluralistic society, assessing the authority of moral consensus in a field such as bioethics involves going beyond political philosophy to the study of actual social processes. An analysis of the nature of representation in an ethics panel's relation to the larger society and its values leads me to reject a legislative model of representation in favor of a deliberative one. After considering the idea that ethical experts might be used to circumvent problems of representation and moral consensus, I conclude with some remarks about my model of ethics panels composed of democratic deliberators.

   Some of the questions addressed in this and the next few chapters are: How can a bioethical consensus be justified in a liberal society that allegedly refrains from dictating the meaning of the "good life"? How can the bioethical consensus that does in fact obtain have legitimate moral authority under such circumstances? What can be learned from studying actual consensus processes, not only in ethics panels in health care but in small groups generally? These questions demand reference to political philosophy and the social sciences. My appeal to material from these disciplines is selective, and neither as complete nor as comprehensive as careful scholarship in these subjects demands; as a philosopher, I am especially aware that my account of political liberalism is a mere sketch. But this is a book about bioethics, not political philosophy or social science, and my purpose is to develop a deeper understanding of moral consensus in bioethics using resources from the basic research that is available.

I have said that bioethics relies on the nexus of autonomy and consensus. In our society individuals are supposed to be free to pursue their own vision of the good life (autonomy) and to enter into common agreements about such a vision (consensus). In this way bioethics participates in the liberal tradition. The classic statement of liberal philosophy is that of John Stuart Mill in *On Liberty*:

The only purpose for which power can be rightfully exercised over any member of a civilized community, against his will, is to prevent harm to others. His own good, either physical or moral, is not a sufficient warrant. He cannot rightfully be compelled to do or forbear because it will be better for him to do so, because it will make him happier, because, in the opinions of others to do so would be wise or even right. These are good reasons for remonstrating with him, or reasoning with him, or persuading him, or entreating him, but not for compelling him, or visiting him with any evil in case he do otherwise.[1]

The idea of the zone of personal autonomy applies also to the power of the state; it constrains the state to neutrality with respect to personal values. The state may not dictate any particular vision of the good life, nor may it use its police power to enforce it. Individuals may join together under the auspices of one or another such conception; indeed, it is thought that these sorts of voluntary arrangements will make for the most vigorous and satisfying civil life. The moral authority of these consensual arrangements derives from the rightful autonomy of the individual, which (according to a view that is deeply embedded in Western philosophy from Aristotle to Kant) is an ethical value that deserves to be respected. The moral authority of any consensus that results from these arrangements is therefore derived from the intrinsic moral status of the autonomous individual. Even if a particular group's own consensus does not reflect that of the larger society, so long as that subgroup respects the general principles of liberalism, its view of the good life is entitled to respect. This is the essence of the political rationale for the authority of consensus in a liberal society.

Again, according to the political rationale, a subgroup's consensus may not infringe on the right of individuals to live in accord with their own comprehensive vision of the good life, even if those conceptions vary greatly from one another. Personal autonomy is the fundamental value of the liberal society in the sense that freedom and equality can be derived from it, but not the reverse. In a diverse or "multicultural" society this substantive liberal value gives subgroups the freedom to pursue their own particularized substantive moral consensus, and each of them must in turn grant that freedom to other groups. Liberals believe that this should pose no insuperable obstacles to social peace. In Max Charlesworth's formulation, "It is possible to have a society without any substantive agreement or consensus on basic moral and religious values."[2]

But surely differences will still arise in practice, differences that must be ameliorated for a complex, modern society to function. In a society that is both liberal and pluralist in its values, how are differences to be overcome without some shared principles beyond that of respect for personal autonomy? The classical view is austere in this regard: the only standards the state may legitimately impose are those that allow for the peaceable resolution of differences in the course of protecting the individual's freedom to pursue his or her own vision of the good life. From this there follows only certain fairly abstract principles that are meant to ensure a respect for freedom and equality, as contrasted with some relatively specific principles that favor one vision of the good life over others.

My purpose is to sketch the political rationale for the authority of consensus that is afforded by the framework of liberal philosophy, not to provide a comprehensive presentation and defense of that philosophy. Nonetheless, at least two sorts of problems have been advanced by critics of the doctrine of liberal neutrality which have special relevance to the basis of moral consensus. First, it is argued that the liberal state is not in fact a "level playing field" on which different views of the good life are respected, for the state itself has interests that it seeks to advance. The idea that the state has an interest in the continuing life of its citizens, for example, is one that can be found in Aristotle and that has played an important role in bioethical debates about decisions to forgo life-sustaining treatment, especially in incompetent patients.

To take an example, gravely ill children whose parents hold religious beliefs concerning therapies which are not scientifically validated are regarded as entitled to scientific medical treatment against their parents' will on the grounds that a child has not yet achieved the capacity to decide in an autonomous manner to associate with those religious beliefs. A familiar example is the choice of prayer rather than chemotherapy for a child who is afflicted with a treatable leukemia. The state's approach ranks beneficence toward the child, and secondarily the protection and promotion of the child's potential autonomy, above other values such as parental authority or the tenets of a particular religious faith. It also provides a basis for the charge that classical liberalism views social life as essentially a contingent conjunction of atomistic individuals. (Although I do not subscribe to this view in general, it may be cogent as a criticism of more extreme versions of libertarianism.) Thus, the first criticism of the doctrine of liberal neutrality is that in practice the liberal state is not truly neutral with regard to all basic values.

The question whether the doctrine of liberal neutrality is a viable conception of the state is important for the idea of a national ethics commission because without it the commission could be seen merely and inevitably as a manifestation of state interests, including the interests of powerful groups with special access to political authorities. On this view, its moral consensus could be wholly reduced to political consensus. Ethics committees, while local both in origin and in their concern with institutional policies and cases, are theoretically subject to some of the same constraints as ethics commissions in their search for shared values and principles. In particular health care institutions, local political forces could hold sway over processes that are advertised as open and candid. When these factors are considered, it becomes clear that the validity of moral consensus is at hazard from many sources.

Many health care institutions, however, are also the products of private associations, and so they are entitled to express particular values that represent consensual views of the good life. This is precisely what is meant by "private," for these are voluntary partnerships of individuals. Hence the "voluntary hospital." Under these conditions, it might be argued, one is entitled to expect only that particular institutions in a liberal society will subscribe to the most general moral principles that would be assumed by society's members properly to apply to those institutions. If that were the case, then the "social contract" would validate the mechanisms that these institutions have devised in order to advance their respective missions so long as they were consistent with those generally assumed principles, and among these mechanisms would be ethics committees. For example, hospitals that operate under the jurisdiction of a particular ecclesiastical authority are entitled to establish policies that express the values inherent in that association. But they are also expected to honor the rights of individuals to decide whether they can accept those values that may affect their care as patients. Thus, institutional policies that follow from these values must be announced in advance.

Since it is not my aim to examine the idea of the self-interested liberal state, my reaction to it is a pragmatic one. I take it that occasions when the state seeks to advance its interests will be perceptible. Therefore, what is required at a minimum is a readiness to scrutinize consensus processes; recall the prize for which we pay the fee of eternal vigilance. Later I will have more to say about the importance of scrutinizing actual consensus processes.

A second sort of criticism of the doctrine of liberal neutrality is not that it is a facade but that it is genuine. As a result, liberalism is unable to give persistent validation to any particular vision of the good life, or even to justify a consensus about some aspect or other of that which is said to be the good life. It is basically a formalistic doctrine that creates a public space but no binding ties. Since liberalism can offer no principled vision of the good life, liberal societies that are faced with a plurality of beliefs are doomed to endless cycles of inconclusive debates about issues such as the termination of life-sustaining treatment and the distribution of health care resources. Because any one conception of the good life is as valid as any other, consensus can be at best a fleeting association with no foundation. On this account, since liberal society cannot validate a particular substantive moral consensus (beyond its fundamental but abstract value of personal autonomy), it therefore provides no basis for explaining why the rest of us should "buy into" the moral consensus of a number of members of society, such as an ethics panel.

Thus, according to Emanuel, a consensus about medical ethics should provide "substantive guidance" to physicians in various situations rather than merely delineate decision-making procedures according to abstract rights. And even when rights are invoked, he contends, the result is either vapid (the idea of "substituted judgment" is one of his examples) or inconclusive (such as the empty slogan of a "right to health care"). He traces these failures to the notion that the liberal state is constrained by its neutrality from identifying a single view of the ends of human life.[3]

This second criticism of the doctrine of liberal neutrality might not pose a problem for societal subgroups, cultures within which there is consensus about more elaborate ethical principles. If there are communities of affected persons who do in fact subscribe to the same ethical principles (including agreement about who has the authority to interpret and implement them), then the consensus of ethics committees in the institutions that serve those individuals under the rubric of an articulated mission is thus legitimated. This might turn out to be true, say, in Roman Catholic hospitals that serve patients who can be presumed to subscribe to specific Roman Catholic ethical principles and who are prepared to submit to ecclesiastical authority.

Yet there is no denying that this criticism is troubling in its implications for ethics committees in most health care institutions, not to mention government ethics commissions in a multicultural society. Consider the ethnic and cultural pluralism that characterizes so many of our inner-city medical centers. Consensus on more highly ramified ethical principles, as contrasted with relatively abstract ones such as the peaceable resolution of differences, might well turn out to be unreliable. Here I have in mind data such as those suggesting that African-American and Hispanic patients have somewhat different attitudes toward the abatement of life-sustaining treatment from white patients.[4] If consensus about more ramified principles among all those concerned is taken as the moral basis for the authority of an ethics committee's consensus, then it is hard to see how a committee can ever arrive at any contentful recommendations under those circumstances.

Thus it appears that many specific elements of the contemporary bioethical consensus is at hazard in our liberal society. Surely this gives us reason to doubt the validity of consensus reached by ethics panels outside of monocultural settings. It would seem that either all the allegedly consensus-based conclusions of modern bioethics and its organs have no moral authority in a pluralistic environment when they have even minimal content (with the exception of panels authorized by and serving monocultural groups), or we must find some way of supplementing Millian liberalism. In a sense this challenge to the idea of moral consensus based on liberal philosophical principles sets the agenda for the remainder of this book.

Again, according to liberal political philosophy the state is not permitted to authorize a particularized moral consensus. Individuals, however, are free to join together to endorse particular principles, even though the reasons they give for doing so may vary. That this may occur in spite of the lack of a deep consensus is the dearest hope of a pluralistic society. I believe that this has in fact occurred in the case of many of the propositions of modern bioethics. What is needed is a device that can conveniently characterize the latent possibility of a valid consensus, even on elaborate moral principles, in a liberal and pluralistic society.

The idea of an overlapping consensus

The political philosopher John Rawls has been concerned in his writings with the achievement by pluralistic and democratic societies of what he calls an "overlapping consensus." It is an elaboration of two ideas that are companions to his central idea of justice as fairness, "of society as a fair system of cooperation over time, from one generation to the next."[5] The first companion idea is that of citizens cooperating as free and equal persons. The second is that of a society regulated by a political conception of justice, a well-ordered society. These ideas could then gain the support of an overlapping consensus, which includes not only those in concert but also

all the reasonable opposing religious, philosophical, and moral doctrines likely to persist over generations and to gain a sizable body of adherents in a more or less constitutional regime, a regime in which that criterion of justice is the political conception itself.[6]

Rawls is interested in finding a basis for social peace in a constitutional democracy that is not only a fragile Hobbesian political agreement nor a mere cease-fire in a war of all against all, but a standard or set of standards that is stable over generations and not merely the temporary result of an ad hoc negotiating process. A framework that includes even opposing doctrines of the good can be the object of an overlapping consensus so long as the regime is just, when a just regime is understood as ensuring the fair treatment of individuals. In this way political institutions should be justifiable so that citizens will have a sincere allegiance to them rather than only acquiesce to state power. It is apparent that these two desiderata— fair treatment of individuals and justifiable institutions—are complementary.

We might say that say that Rawls is interested in how stability might be forged in a society that is both liberal and diverse. Deep consensus is not required for the political morality Rawls envisions. Rather, what is required is that all groups will be equally free to pursue their vision of the good life and continue to endorse those institutions and principles that ensure that they can do so. In Rawls's account the principle of justice as fairness is to be thought of as the object of an overlapping consensus. I contend that other, more ramified principles, such as those found in bioethics, may also be objects of an overlapping consensus.

Consider, for example, the four principles usually included in the bioethics mantra: justice, autonomy, nonmaleficence, and beneficence. Justice is already inscribed in the overlapping consensus as fairness; autonomy, understood as entailing freedom and equality, is a prerequisite to the political conception of justice; nonmaleficence may be viewed as jointly implied by a respect for free and equal persons entitled to fair treatment; and beneficence is a more contentful expression of that respect. Thus, to honor someone's autonomy is to give that person what he or she deserves, as those who are ill may reasonably expect that health care professionals will attempt to benefit them insofar as that is consistent with the other principles. The principles become more highly articulated as they refer to more highly ramified states of affairs, but it would be arbitrary to specify a point at which procedural principles end and substantive principles begin. That competent patients may decline life-sustaining treatment is, among other things, a specification of the principle of autonomy, a principle that also helps justify the more articulate one about competent patients.[7] The exact principles that are the objects of an overlapping consensus, and the extent to which they are more or less articulate, depends to a great extent on the context in which they are being entertained.

In something like this way, some bioethical principles can be the enduring objects of an overlapping consensus. There are, however, certain principles that may not achieve this status but will always be controversial. An example is that concerning a woman's right to an abortion late in pregnancy. To succeed, an overlapping consensus must include these more or less predictable and stable disagreements in a system that promises significant stability by including all those "reasonable opposing religious, philosophical, and moral doctrines likely to persist over generations." In other words, the opposing and persistent doctrines must be held in a relatively stable tension within the framework of the overlapping consensus. Now, of course we have societal controversies that are too highly ramified to be satisfied by the mere recitation of the abstract principle of justice—moral controversies that can be divisive. These controversies require management in ways that are reasonable and with which the citizenry can identify. Bioethics concerns itself with many such controversies. Because it deals with relatively novel problems and cases, and because it demands of consensus-based principles that they deal with quite specific factual situations, bioethics is the kind of practice that places a strain on the political rationale for the authority of consensus in a liberal and pluralistic society.

The political rationale for consensus appears to reach its limit here, for the endurance of an overlapping consensus that includes the reasonable opposing doctrines likely to persist over generations seems to place an extraordinary burden on the *processes* of moral consensus. They must be regarded as honoring the values that are held in a stable balance within the framework of overlapping consensus. Thus, while an overlapping consensus must not only protect against a patently invalid consensus, such as that which undergirded Nazi eugenics, by respecting the freedom and equality of all, it must also develop satisfactory mechanisms for the management of reasonable and persistent disagreements. This is especially difficult because, unlike in the case of protecting a minority from exploitation, these mechanisms also have to address certain positive actions, such as the implementation of government policy to provide abortions to those who wish them while also respecting the views of those who are deeply opposed to such a policy. In much of the rest of this book I will be concerned with the problem of extending a valid moral consensus in a liberal and diverse society, a problem that forces us to look beyond the political rationale to actual consensus processes.

Extending moral consensus

We should pause to remind ourselves why the extension of moral consensus in a diverse, pluralistic society is an especially important matter for bioethics. Unlike traditional medical ethics, which was mainly concerned with codifying certain ideals of physician conduct, modern bioethics trades in controversial subjects that are of broad interest to the polity. Entities within the institution of bioethics, and especially ethics panels, have been given the job of finding ways to accommodate extant values to novel states of affairs. The specific problem that concerns us is how these panels can hope to pursue the valid extension of the overlapping consensus in a liberal, pluralistic society. Only recently have writers in bioethics taken seriously the importance of process, an emphasis that is akin to my own.[8]

It is easy to see what difficulties this matter of extending moral consensus presents for ethics panels, even those guided by principles that are among the objects of an overlapping consensus. Ethics commissions and committees must somehow produce decisions or recommendations that are valid expressions of moral consensus in a pluralistic society. But how can the consensus-based conclusions of such panels be reasonably assured of enjoying a valid moral authority?

We have returned by a circuitous route to the second criticism of liberalism, for another way of stating the problem is this: even if we suppose that a certain set of rather abstract principles can be the object of an overlapping consensus, in practice decisions are going to have to be made that are relatively specific to content and that do not strictly follow from those principles. Often they will be made by small groups of people, such as ethics panels. Inevitably some members of the polity, or even most, are not going to subscribe to some of the decisions that have supposedly been made under the rubric of the principles in the overlapping consensus. Yet it is possible to assert justifiably, in at least some cases, that these panels' conclusions have moral authority. How can the liberal society accept such a result?

The answer to this important question is that, in general, so long as the small group's particularized consensus upholds liberal values such as respect for the personal autonomy of those who disagree and a willingness to consider alternative points of view, then the panel's consensus has all the moral authority that a deliberative process can be accorded in a liberal society. Liberalism does not require of a small group of decision makers that they agree with the society in detail, but it does demand accord with the general conditions that govern the conduct of this kind of process. Yet the panel's particularized moral consensus may not be imposed on individuals in such a way that it interferes with their rightful personal autonomy.

How can we know when these conditions have been satisfied? Only, I would argue, by paying case-by-case attention to the processes according to which consensus-based panels operate. Lacking unambiguous justification by authoritative principles, a panel's consensus about a particular state of affairs depends crucially on the qualities of the process from which that consensus emerged. These qualities must respect basic liberal values—values that are expressed in principles that are among the objects of an overlapping consensus, such as mutual respect, openness to alternative points of view, and willingness to entertain unpopular views. Another value that must be reflected in these processes is the consideration of relevant factual information, an important part of what John Dewey called "social intelligence." Thus, we will shortly be led to the study of consensus processes in ethics panels, in health care, and in small groups generally. But unless we go beyond what I have called the political rationale to the study of the way these qualities may or may not appear in actual consensus processes, we will not really have taken seriously the practical problems associated with the authority of consensus in a field such as bioethics.

Since the principles that are the objects of an overlapping consensus do not strictly imply certain conclusions in particular cases of moral consensus, they cannot be mechanically applied to specific cases. This "engineering" model of bioethical analysis has been rightly discredited.[9] Rawls has coined the term "reflective equilibrium" to refer to the optimal balance between principles and considered judgments. The understanding of the principles that are the objects of an overlapping consensus is engaged in a continual give and take with judgments about the ethical issues with which panels are confronted. Each undergoes continual modification in light of the other. At some point the mutual modification of ethical principle and moral judgment reaches a complementary balance.[10]

In extending a moral consensus into new and controversial territory, we open ourselves up to the problem that values may be less stable than is desirable from the standpoint of the overlapping consensus. For instance, until the diverse members of the liberal polity are comfortable with the idea that artificial hydration and nutrition is a life-sustaining treatment that may be forgone if the patient or appropriate surrogate insists, the values underlying this highly articulated principle of clinical ethics will be unstable. Nevertheless, to the extent that a panel's process has respected more general liberal values, their conclusion will possess a degree of moral authority. Again, to a great extent the stability of emerging principles will depend on the degree to which the process from which they emerge is in accord with certain values that are uncontroversial in a liberal society. I have argued that these uncontroversial standards would include nonviolent methods, mutual respect, and a willingness to entertain new evidence and alternative points of view. These are standards that are themselves objects of an overlapping consensus in a liberal, pluralistic society. So when we assess the extension of a more or less settled moral consensus, we might well inquire first as to whether those principles that *do* apply, however modest they may be, are actually honored in the process.

By studying actual consensus processes we can learn more about how the qualities we should be able to expect of deliberation in ethics panels manifest themselves. This is a study that bioethics must take up not only because of the limitations of the political rationale for the authority of consensus, but also because bioethics is both an academic field and a movement engaged in social change. Whatever the precise details of the qualities that validate an ethics panel's consensus process, the "stretch" of a panel's interpretation of a principle beyond what was precisely intended by the society's moral consensus is often an important facet of a panel's mission. Since the society as a whole cannot be expected to consider each new case or problem, some subset of members of the society must do so. Indeed, this social need is exactly the reason why many practices in the institution of bioethics exist, including review by individual ethics consultants as well as panels, so that there is some systematic effort to weigh and, if needed, extend the consensus of a pluralistic and technologically innovative society. The aim of the overlapping consensus—to provide an enduring framework even among those reasonable and persistent disagreements—will be satisfied only to the extent that this extension can be accomplished.

In the course of their work the members of an ethics panel may find not only that the understanding of principles that are among the objects of a societal consensus must be extended, but also that this proposal must be communicated to the wider society, especially when the panel's consensus is not likely to be popular, or when it deals with novel cases or problems. In fact, education is an essential part of the business of preserving the framework of an overlapping consensus. On this view, part of the obligation of the panel is to educate the society about its findings. This education will, of course, take various forms, depending on the circumstances. Ethics commissions are naturally expected to issue a report, and ethics committees must "report out" their findings to the protagonists in the case, to hospital authorities, and perhaps to the institution's staff in the form of a conference or grand rounds.

There is an obvious and welcome analogy here to the way the legal system extends precedent as novel nuances are encountered in particular cases. It is reasonable to expect both that the spirit of the set of precedents will be extended but not distorted, and that the process will be one that respects due process. One reason why the courts exist is to play this role with regard to the extension of legal principles. And the courts educate the society formally through court reports and de facto through the media and other public organs. But the analogy is not perfect because, unlike in the legal system, the values that are the object of the consensus in a pluralistic society are usually not so clearly expressed. A possible exception is the common law, which might be regarded as part of the societal consensus. In any case, this difference between the legal system and the extension of the overlapping consensus places a special burden on the way certain individuals are "chosen" to represent the pluralistic society in ethics panels. It also indicates that the process by which the extension of the societal consensus is effected, the preservation of the framework of overlapping consensus, is far murkier than is the case in the legal system. The murkiness of moral consensus processes, and the evolution of the overlapping consensus, is another good reason for subjecting those processes to empirical examination, as I shall do in subsequent chapters.

In this chapter I have been concerned with the question how a moral consensus can be valid in a liberal and diverse society. Some may assert that, even if consensus can be achieved with regard to relatively contentful ethical problems, this does not settle the question whether such a consensus is "right" in a transcendental sense. That is, it does not settle the question whether a societal consensus is morally right as well as politically acceptable. Now, according to liberal political philosophy this assertion misses the point, for there is an irreducibly moral element in the political rationale, one that is expressed in political terms as freedom and equality. According to liberal philosophers, so long as these conditions are respected, it is pointless to demand more of the political system and insist on a transcendental standard of morality. This is not to say that political processes that meet the requirements of liberalism will automatically result in morally sound conclusions; rather, we can proceed with the assessment of those conclusions by determining whether they have satisfied the requirements of liberalism. Nor is it to say that some within the political system will not appeal to transcendental moral standards, but only that such appeals are not decisive in the liberal society.

One may argue that the liberal political rationale for the authority of consensus has not truly joined the issue in its response to the charge of amorality, a question to which I return in chapter 7. In any case, there are clearly many issues in bioethics that cannot be conclusively resolved by attention to the demands of political philosophy alone, for these demands are minimal and are not designed to aid in developing a detailed moral consensus. Thus, the question whether a retarded child should serve as a kidney donor for the sake of a "normal" sibling may be one around which a certain legal and social consensus forms in favor of such a measure.[11] Further reflection could eventuate in the determination that the procedure does not sufficiently respect the freedom and equality of the donor. In this case, the liberal requirement that he or she be accorded this respect was at least partially satisfied by the fact that due process of law was engaged, but a later consensus could emerge to the effect that the respect embodied in the process was not enough. Liberalism accords to moral controversy the potential for extending its principles by consensus, but it cannot reasonably be expected to dictate their interpretation beyond a certain point. Apart from large-scale societal consensus, public confidence in the consensus-based conclusions of ethics panels requires a confidence in the quality of the deliberators as well as in their deliberative processes, and especially in terms of the composition of panel membership.

The problem of representation

Diversity of representation is normally thought to be an essential feature of ethics panels in a diverse liberal, democratic society. But what is meant by representation here? We do not normally think that criteria for membership on an ethics panel must achieve the formal status required of standards for the judge in a court of law. Nor do we even require that commission or committee members endure the scrutiny imposed on candidates for a jury, though there is a suggestive similarity in the principle that one's peers are likely to represent the values of the wider community that is symbolically passing judgment. Rather, we tend to assume that the members of an ethics panel will find a way to extend or in some way satisfy the conditions implicit in the society's overlapping consensus, or that they will do so to the greatest extent possible, however we construe the nature of that consensus.

And yet panel members are often selected because the issues to be considered involve technical matters (medical, legal, social, or philosophical ones) that make it wise to include "experts." Furthermore, many ethics committees stipulate the membership of a "community representative," presumably to ensure that technical values do not predominate, and also to help diversify the moral values represented in the committee's deliberations. As we shall see, this is also recommended for ethics commissions. According to the theoretical framework I have been developing, this measure can be understood as an attempt by a liberal society to extend its relatively stable and predictable overlapping consensus. Although the criteria for membership on an ethics panel are far looser than for a jury, it is clear that what is sought for the panel as a whole is that it will represent the diverse views that participate in the overlapping consensus.

The language of representation can be misleading, for an ethics panel is not a moral legislature. Ethics panel members represent the wider society in a deliberative rather than in a legislative sense. Thus they neither simply represent the views of "constituents" nor necessarily express themselves by their voting. Yet in order to influence the consensus that might finally be reached by the wider community from which they are drawn, they must have value dispositions reasonably similar to those of the community. One obvious problem with this account is that it fails to address the possibility that the shared values might nonetheless be venal. Recall, however, the basis of a liberal society, which respects the personal autonomy of its members. This is not to suggest that the liberal framework can guarantee that the intentions of its members toward one another will always be kind and gentle, but only that when they are vicious, they are constrained by limitations on conduct. The goal of liberalism is not to reform personal character but to monitor public action.

Even when the intentions of members of the liberal polity are not self-consciously venal, they may be wrongheaded. This is where the rough distinction between substantive and procedural values is useful. As in the famous case of the Seattle kidney dialysis selection committee, sometimes prejudices inherent in substantive values are exposed in a way that conflicts with liberal procedural values, even to a degree that embarrasses the panel itself. Thus it might be argued that both the inequities of its recommendations and its realization of these inequities were dispositions to be found within the society. Hence the society was ultimately able to accept and identify with the self-criticism of the selection committee.

Still, Pollyanna has no place in matters as grave as these. The example seems to suggest that a body of democratic deliberators should represent the more general and abstract value consensus of the wider community while guarding against the uncritical embrace of its more specific values. Again, gathering the facts, hearing from concerned parties, considering the wisdom of relevant extant policies, respecting the civil rights and moral agency of those involved, and willingly entertaining reasonable appeals all count as manifestations of consensus-based values. Yet the fact that the community has apparently embraced a particular point of view is information with respect to which the panel should be prepared to take a critical stand. Of course it is practically (and perhaps logically) impossible for all of the more contentful societal values to be bracketed, but the ethics panel must be prepared to view any particular assumption, no matter how widely held, with a degree of philosophical detachment. Still more difficult, though perhaps at least as important, is for the panel to be prepared to view itself and its processes with a similar critical detachment.

There is a specific aspect of the problem of representation that is typical of panels in bioethics because such a field marries technical and moral issues. An example of this problem can be gleaned from the IRB experience. Robert Veatch has observed that to meet their mandate, IRBs have included members with professional skills who are able to evaluate technical proposals. But IRBs are also expected to be able to judge community attitudes; thus they must have members with representative skills. While the former members must be possessed of professional expertise, the latter are to be chosen according to their approximation of the criterion of the "typical reasonable person." The absence of either will alter the committee's conclusions, but a mixed committee will be hard put to reflect the community because professionals tend to have certain socioeconomic characteristics and values, thus skewing the conclusions. One solution Veatch recommends, somewhat reluctantly, is a dual committee system for research in which the professionals establish scientific merit and the lay people the community standards.[12]

Ethics committees do not as yet operate under the sort of legal mandate that holds for IRBs. But just as scientific merit is a legitimate consideration when an IRB considers a research protocol, so the medical merit of an intervention is often a legitimate consideration for an ethics committee. Yet no serious commentator, so far as I know, has called for an ethics committee that wholly excludes professional expertise. Nor do I believe that such a committee could possibly be efficacious in influencing clinical practices in an institution beyond the immediate case. Rather, most seem to think that the combination of professional experts and "typical reasonable people" can be embodied in a single committee. Perhaps this is easier to accomplish in an ethics committee than in an IRB because in the former only therapies that already meet the standard of practice are being considered, so the requisite degree of scientific expertise is less.

Before moving on I want to say a word about the "typical reasonable person" criterion itself. This standard falls short, but not because it is vague. Actually it is quite specific, perhaps even empirically supportable, although unavoidably general. It falls short because one would like to know more about the underlying conditions that enable anyone to be typical in the relevant sense. My own answer to this question, to be elaborated later, combines the data of empirical psychology and the generalizations of moral psychology. Put in quasi-behavioral terms, chances are that someone randomly chosen from our society is disposed to respond in ways that lead inexorably around that web of societal values (albeit with individual differences of expression and emphasis), and does so both without knowing it and without being able to avoid it. This raises a question about how moral consensus can be explained in a psychological sense. What follows anticipates a lengthier presentation in chapter 7.

In the history of moral philosophy the eighteenth-century Scottish philosopher Francis Hutcheson is particularly identified with the view that a moral sense exists. According to Hutcheson, just as the physical senses of sight and hearing inform our physical judgments, so is there a sense that informs our moral judgments.[13] There is nothing "supernatural" about this moral sense. The judgments to which it is related are just as natural and common as those of vision. Judgments of benevolence, for example, are derived through objective perceptions that are largely shared by humanity. Those who lack the capacity to arrive at these judgments are impaired, as are those who lack the capacity to arrive at physical judgments.

Although some features of Hutcheson's philosophy were rejected by other important Scottish philosophers, including Adam Smith[14] and David Hume,[15] his work enjoyed a residual influence. In particular Smith and Hume agreed that, however it is described, there is something about human beings that enables them to express virtually universal agreement on basic moral propositions. There is in this tradition an implicit, empirically based philosophy of moral consensus that I want to recapture. I expand on the idea of a naturalized theory of consensus in chapter 8.

Ethics experts and democratic deliberation

Some individuals who are recruited to serve on ethics panels are selected precisely because they are considered to be "ethics experts." If there were ethics experts, we wouldn't need to worry about representation, or even consensus, since we could just put our moral quandaries in their hands. Nor would we need to wonder how consensus achieves moral authority. There is a generic paradox in the relation between the ideas of ethical expertise and consensus, since one might well suppose that experts in any field should always agree, but the brute fact is that they do not, whether in science or ethics. The idea that true experts should always agree probably derives from Plato, according to whom the philosopher-kings could not disagree about the Good because it is undivided and they would all have the same access to it. On further consideration, however, we find no obvious reason why experts should not disagree and still be worthy of the title, especially about novel problems that require the extension of their store of knowledge and information.

A similar point is made by Ellen Fox and Carol Stocking in their study of ethics consultants' recommendations:

It would not be uncommon for two well-respected infectious disease specialists consulting on the same patient to disagree on the optimal combination of antibiotics. Few would regard such a disagreement as material evidence for a lack of expertise on the part of either specialist. Instead, such disagreements are commonly considered matters of style. Analogously, then, ethics consultants might also be allowed a certain latitude in their recommendations.[16]

Nevertheless, these writers express sensible concern that the ethics consultants they surveyed diverged greatly in their recommendations about several case scenarios. Unlike the goal in the medical specialty of infectious disease, where there can be agreement about desirable outcomes and eventually about which therapies are the most likely to produce such outcomes, the goal of ethics consultation is itself a controversial matter. Fox and Stocking conclude that, if the plan of ethics organizations "is to achieve consensus among ethics consultants, they may have a formidable task ahead of them."[17] Left open in this formulation is the possibility that delineating a range of acceptable alternatives is an acceptable goal for ethics panels, though even that strategy does not obviate a role for consensus.

Indeed, similar observations can be made concerning ethics panels that reach different conclusions about similar cases even though they are similarly constituted from one institution to the next and follow similar procedures. How can the theoretical framework I have developed account for this situation? I believe the answer is not that the societal consensus can be stretched too far and torn, for there are always going to be some principles of minimal content to which all panels can subscribe in any given case, even if they are "only" procedural ones. Rather, I would say that new ethics cases and problems introduce details that we cannot confidently associate with existing understandings of the principles that are among the objects of the overlapping consensus. Eventually we should be able to do so, but only after an extended social conversation about the troubling cases, a conversation that will take place in part within ethics panels and among groups of ethics experts.

In the meantime, if we are to preserve as much of the stability of the overlapping consensus as possible, the integrity of the process must be jealously guarded. To do this, ethics panel members and ethics experts will need to understand the nature of consensus processes. Thus, again, there is a manifest need for bioethics to study moral consensus processes, especially in small groups. My more general account of moral consensus processes regards panel members as democratic deliberators.

Emanuel has written about the role of democratic deliberation in bioethics. He argues that democratic political procedures require "collective practical reasoning," a setting of "free and equal persons collectively participating in self-rule and, through it, self-development."[18] His model is that archetype of direct democratic deliberation and self-rule, the New England town meeting. Collectives of not more than 25,000 people, he contends, could engage in this kind of interaction and establish health care institutions that in their policies would conform to a shared vision of the good life. Each "community health program" (CHP) would enjoy a philosophical framework to guide policies, one settled upon by the collective to guide decisions about what sorts of care to provide.

Emanuel's proposal is reminiscent of the "community consultation" model that was exemplified most famously in the state of Oregon in 1987, when many citizens were asked whether basic health services should be provided to three thousand disadvantaged Oregonians if that meant eliminating the organ transplant program that benefited about thirty people. The reflective responses were incorporated into the proposed revision of the state's Medicaid regulations.[19]

This project, like Emanuel's proposal, falls into a tradition in recent liberal political philosophy that can be associated with John Dewey. Dewey was strongly influenced by town meeting democracy, and his idea of social intelligence is closely akin to that of collective practical reasoning. So long as the personal autonomy of the members of the community is respected, liberalism can endorse these kinds of consensual arrangements by subgroups. In this sense community consultation is arguably a requirement of liberal democracy, so that the members of the polity have the opportunity to express themselves on substantive moral questions, the answers to which are certain to affect them.[20]

An ethics panel's conclusions, however, need not square with the popular view in order to have moral authority in a liberal society. At the same time, their highly articulated conclusions cannot be validly imposed on the private affairs of those who hold different moral values that are themselves consistent with the most general principles of liberal society (though there will always be vigorous debates about the meaning and extent of privacy); to do so jeopardizes the framework of the overlapping consensus. The consensus processes of panels engaged in moral

deliberation in a liberal and democratic society are not "legislative" but deliberative, for, as we have seen, they cannot impose, much less presuppose, a vision of
the good life. The force of their deliberations is persuasive, exactly the point made
by the proponents of ethics commissions. The ultimate decision of the Oregon
legislature to end reimbursement for organ transplantation under Medicaid was
precisely a legislative decision, albeit one partly arrived at through a process of
democratic deliberation thought by community proponents not to violate liberal
principles because that decision did not interfere with the personal autonomy or
privacy of the affected individuals, who had no entitlement to public funds for
access to organ transplants. This interpretation of the demands of liberalism was,
of course, hotly contested by its critics.

Some aspects of the work done by ethics commissions fall within the idea of
democratic consultation. Ethics committees, too, often cannot presuppose common values in their institutions, but the results of their deliberations will have force
only if they help to forge an institutional consensus. This wider form of deliberative democracy has to involve not only health care professionals but also the communities of patients for whom they are responsible.[21]

It is worth noting parenthetically that the consensus processes I have been describing are of a kind that might be called dynamic, as compared with the static
consensus that can be perceived in the results of a public opinion survey. Only
dynamic consensus makes possible the self-discovery and transformation that is
part of full-blooded consensus processes. Static consensus is useful to policymakers
who want to avoid introducing legislation that is doomed to failure and political
figures who wish to solicit votes. True leadership takes the far riskier course of
immersion in dynamic consensus processes. And yet, beyond the political rationale for the authority of moral consensus which I have reconstructed in this chapter, dynamic consensus processes invoke the ambiguities and uncertainties of the
world as it is.

Notes

1. John Stuart Mill, *On Liberty*, ed. R. B. McCullum (Oxford: Basil Blackwell, 1946),
   pp. 8–9.
2. Max Charlesworth, *Bioethics in a Liberal Society* (Cambridge: Cambridge University Press, 1993), p. 18.
3. Emanuel, *Ends of Human Life*, p. 19.
4. P. V. Caralis et al., "The Influence of Ethnicity and Race on Attitudes Toward Advance Directives, Life-Prolonging Treatments, and Euthanasia," *Journal of Clinical
   Ethics* 4, 2 (1993): 155–65.
5. John Rawls, *A Theory of Justice* (Cambridge, Mass.: Harvard University Press, 1971),
   p. 14.
6. John Rawls, "The Idea of an Overlapping Consensus," *Oxford Journal of Legal Studies*
   7, 1 (1981): 15. One criticism of the idea of overlapping consensus is that it illicitly
   introduces the "value" of societal stability, but it is hard to see how one could object

to the treatment of persons as free and equal, and therefore to the stability that could result from the polity's appreciation of this condition.

7. For more on the idea of specified principles, see Henry S. Richardson, "Specifying Norms as a Way to Resolve Concrete Ethics Problems," *Philosophy and Public Affairs* 19, 4 (1990): 279–310; and David DeGrazia, "Moving Forward in Bioethical Theory: Theories, Cases, and Specified Principles," *Journal of Medicine and Philosophy* 17, 5 (1992): 511–39.

8. See Susan M. Wolf, "Toward a Theory of Process," *Journal of Law, Medicine, and Health Care* 20, 4 (1992): 278–90. Wolf argues that process values can include that of being patient-centered (showing respect for the patient by treating her as the central feature of the process) and that of treating different patients equitably (not discriminating). I am in strong agreement with her that explicit discussion and adoption of process values would be salutary for bioethics so as to narrow the gap between the theory of bioethics and clinical practices. Furthermore, as I have argued, even process values are subject to consensus processes, so the nature of consensus must also be part of the bioethical conversation.

9. Arthur L. Caplan, "Can Applied Ethics Be Effective in Health Care and Should It Strive to Be?," in *"If I Were a Rich Man Could I Buy a Pancreas?" and Other Essays on the Ethics of Health Care* (Bloomington: Indiana University Press, 1992), pp. 3–17.

10. Rawls, *Theory of Justice*.

11. The scenario described in this paragraph actually occurred in the case of *Strunk v. Strunk* 445 S.W. 2d 145, Ky. 1969.

12. Veatch, "Consensus of Expertise," p. 442.

13. Francis Hutcheson, *An Essay on the Nature and Conduct of the Passions and Affections, with Illustrations on the Moral Sense*, 3d ed. (Gainesville, Fla.: Scholars' Facsimiles and Reprints, 1969).

14. Adam Smith, *The Theory of Moral Sentiments*, ed. D. D. Raphael and A. L. Mache (Oxford: Clarendon, 1976).

15. David Hume, *A Treatise of Human Nature*, ed. L. A. Selby-Bigge (Oxford: Clarendon, 1978).

16. Fox and Stocking, "Ethics Consultants' Recommendations for Life-Prolonging Treatment of Patients in a Persistent Vegetative State," p. 2581.

17. Ibid.

18. Emanuel, *Ends of Human Life*, p. 148.

19. On the Oregon plan, see generally Charles J. Dougherty et al., Special Supplement, *Hastings Center Report* 21, 3 (1991): S1–16.

20. Several of Dewey's books are relevant to this project. See, for example, John Dewey, *The Public and Its Problems* (Denver: Alan Swallow Press, 1927).

21. In fact, of course, the socially intelligent practices that would make democratic deliberators of the general electorate are few and far between. The political scientist James Fishkin has emphasized the difference between educated public opinion and that which is usually expressed in public opinion polls or at voting booths. His idea for a "national issues convention" calls for four hundred to six hundred randomly chosen citizens to immerse themselves in study, lectures, and discussions and vote for candidates after grilling them. The results might even influence the opinions of the rest of the electorate who did not have the opportunity for this deliberative experience. It is a most Deweyan idea. See James Fishkin, *Democracy and Deliberation: New Directions for Democratic Reform* (New Haven: Yale University Press, 1991).

5

National Ethics Commissions

Consensus panels in medical science

This chapter begins with a brief discussion of consensus panels on nonmoral questions of medical science, a recent practice that demonstrates the importance of consensus on a national scale in the institution of modern medicine. The point is that processes concerning specifically *ethical* questions in medicine take place in a context that is oriented toward consensus even on technical questions. I then turn to two examples of national commissions, the National Commission for the Protection of Human Subjects of Biomedical and Behavioral Research (hereafter the National Commission), and the President's Commission for the Study of Ethical Problems in Medicine and Biomedical and Behavioral Research (the President's Commission). My goals are to assess the role of consensus processes in the history of these commissions, and to ascertain in what respects they succeeded or failed as representations of the prospects for moral consensus on bioethical issues on a national level.

There are, of course, numerous examples of nongovernmental consensus groups in bioethics, including research groups organized by organizations such as the Hastings Center and by professional associations such as the Council on Judicial and Ethical Affairs of the American Medical Association. And there are several examples of state ethics commissions, such as the New York State Governor's Task Force on Life and the Law. I focus on federal ethics commissions because the problems they pose include not only those pertinent to these other categories of ethics commission but also those that touch on governmental issues with a national scope. To be sure, government panels are critically different from nongovernmental bodies in that they play a role as part of a representative democracy.

The importance of consensus in the value system of modern medical science shows itself whenever government agencies or professional organizations assemble panels to provide guidance on controversial technical questions. While relatively few physicians function for very long in "cutting-edge" settings, all are expected to honor the best scientific expertise available in their specialties. In this respect the most significant way collective expert agreement *theoretically* affects the professional lives of American physicians once they enter practice is through the National Institutes of Health (NIH) consensus development conference. (I say "theoretically" because telephone surveys have indicated that only 15 to 20 percent of all physicians can recall hearing about any given NIH consensus conference.)[1]

Nonetheless, the very existence of consensus conferences is important for our purposes insofar as they highlight the value placed on agreement by the scientific community, particularly among those considered experts. As I go on to argue, our society also values consensus, including moral consensus, as expressed by its political institutions. The NIH has sponsored over sixty consensus conferences since 1980, each usually lasting about two and a half days, with the goal of exposing the public and medical practitioners to new and existing technologies about which there is some uncertainty. At the end of the conferences the panelists produce written recommendations or guidelines. Experience strongly suggests that the conferences tend not to achieve a consensus for which there is not already strong support in the literature; thus, rather than breaking new ground, they tend to give an imprimatur to a practice that is already extant in the medical community.[2]

In addition to the value placed on consensus, the other value evidenced by these conferences is that of expertise. But Robert Veatch has observed that expert consensus is deeply enmeshed not only with a body of facts but also with the experts' values relevant to those facts. He further holds that lay people, if they had the necessary scientific expertise, would tend to value facts differently, a claim that, if supportable, would gravely undermine the assumption that consensus conference results can serve justifiably as guidelines for public policy.[3]

My specific concern at the moment, however, is not with the claims that have been made on behalf of consensus conferences but rather with the reception of expert consensus within the medical community as a whole. Cautious as their recommendations tend to be, and distinguished as their panelists usually are, consensus conferences do not appear to command the attention of most practitioners. Their distance from those in the field and the seemingly academic quality of their discussions undermine their ability to capture the imagination of their public. Hence, while practitioners may be prepared to recognize their conclusions as "expert" in a formal sense, most do not find them as compelling as their own clinical experience or, perhaps, the views of local "experts" with whom they frequently interact.

A brief history of governmental commissions

If national consensus conferences on technical biomedical issues have limited influence on actual practice, at least in the short run, no more can be expected of consensus reached by national ethics commissions. Yet the government commission, defined as an official agency or institution headed by a collegial body of commissioners, does play an important role in public policy, which gradually transforms professional practice. LeRoy Walters has traced the ancestry of contemporary ethics commissions to the Royal Commission on Poor Laws (1832–34), the body that proposed reforms in the British welfare system, based partly on empirical investigation. The Royal Commission is only the most famous example of a temporary commission with a limited or ad hoc governmental mandate designed to play a role in policymaking.[4]

In the twentieth-century United States several presidents have had a particular penchant for presidential commissions. Theodore Roosevelt appointed six, including a Country Life Commission that investigated the needs of farm families. With the problem-solving orientation of a trained engineer, Herbert Hoover appointed numerous commissions to bring scientific knowledge to bear on matters of government. In the 1960s and 1970s the commission device was applied to several matters of grave public concern. Two such bodies were the National Advisory Commission on Civil Disorders and the President's Commission on the Assassination of President Kennedy. Other nations have institutionalized standing commissions, such as those in Australia and Canada that recommend reforms in the law.

Social scientists have identified several roles for commissions, including giving added legitimacy to official action, sanctioning delay in government action on a controversial matter or recommending unpopular policies, ensuring that competing interests are represented in policy deliberations through a diverse membership, and building public support for new policies. All of these functions have something to do with consensus, generally either lending public and official recognition to a de facto consensus or contributing to the development of a new consensus. Without entering into detailed discussions of the substance of their work, I examine the experiences of the National Commission and the President's Commission with regard to these consensus-oriented functions.

The National Commission

The National Commission for the Protection of Human Subjects of Biomedical and Behavioral Research issued an important document, usually referred to as "The

Belmont Report," in 1979, five years after its founding by an act of Congress. The report actually grew out of discussions that were held by the commissioners in February 1976 at the Smithsonian Institution's Belmont Center. The coincidence of the decision in *Quinlan* that same year identifies this as a landmark period in the development of bioethical consensus.

The greatest single contribution of the Commission was surely the articulation of three ethical principles, or "general prescriptive judgments," intended to provide an "analytical framework that will guide the resolution of ethical problems arising from research involving human subjects."[5] The principles—respect for persons, beneficence, and justice—each represents the essence of long-standing moral traditions; they did not, of course, suddenly spring from the heads of the commissioners, nor even mainly from the history of medical ethics. Beneficence and its sibling nonmaleficence are closely associated with the Hippocratic tradition and in medical research ethics (through the philosophy of Claude Bernard), but they gain their overall legitimacy from the Judaeo-Christian tradition. Respect for persons arguably has roots in classical consensus theory (the consent of the governed), but it gained a firmer foothold in the Enlightenment. The Nuremberg Code asserted the importance of respect for persons in the form of the "voluntary consent of the subject" as its first principle, though other codes, including even a 1931 German Interior Ministry document, expressed the necessity of respecting individual human subjects.[6] And the understanding of justice as equity is familiar from Aristotle and the legal canons he helped found.

It is thus clear that the three Belmont principles, while elegant and useful in their simplicity, were part of an evolution of moral thought from various quarters, part of an exceedingly complex cultural tapestry of moral consensus. Driven by repeated scandals that undermined the credibility of medical research as a humanistic activity, the Commission forcefully insisted that the process of attaining new knowledge is not excluded from the lineaments of moral traditions. In short, the commissioners *theoretically* concluded that there is such a thing as "forbidden knowledge," even that which would in some sense be of great benefit to humankind. My qualification is based on the fact that the National Commission did not specifically rule out utilitarian calculations of risk and benefit in all cases.

With the publication of their influential textbook *The Principles of Biomedical Ethics*, Tom L. Beauchamp (who had been a member of the Commission's professional staff) and James F. Childress brought the three principles into bioethical analysis more generally, with at least one significant alteration: "respect for persons" was more narrowly construed as autonomy, which appears to admit of fewer exceptions. The principles have been wildly successful as conveying the essence of bioethical thought, so much so that they are often referred to somewhat derisively as the "bioethics mantra." As a study in the sociology of knowledge, the evolution of the bioethics mantra reverses what is thought to be the normal relationship between the academic and policymaking worlds, with the former spinning theories that are adopted by the latter and modified to suit political realities. In this case a government commission provided the occasion for the formulation of consensus ethical principles that became the basis for much of the theoretical foundation of an academic field.[7]

Now to the process behind the Commission's discussions. Earlier I mentioned Stephen Toulmin's view that the commissioners reached consensus on specific judgments in individual cases. I have already noted Toulmin's assertion, from his vantage point as a philosopher-consultant to the Commission, that the members did not reach agreement by way of deduction from moral philosophical axioms, and that if they had looked to their more general underlying philosophies, they might well have found themselves in disagreement. To use a term I introduced earlier, according to Toulmin their consensus was not "deep." This account is corroborated by Albert Jonsen, another senior bioethicist who also observed the National Commission, and together they use it to buttress their well-known casuistic approach to ethical issues, as opposed to a more standard "top-down" or deductive appeal to principles.[8]

Interestingly, the two authors who are most closely identified with the methodology of justificatory principles, Beauchamp and Childress, have directly disputed the conclusions Jonsen and Toulmin reach about the National Commission's processes. They note that the transcripts of Commission proceedings show a repeatedly dialectical pattern, as cases that favored one point of view or another were brought up and principles were modified in light of those cases; or at other times cases were dropped owing to the implications of a principle. They conclude that Jonsen and Toulmin have confused *principles* with *theories*, and that in practical terms one could do without ethical theories but not without justificatory principles.[9]

Which side is right in this controversy? In his retrospective assessment of the President's Commission's processes, its executive director, Alexander Morgan Capron, uses terms that are almost identical to those Toulmin used in describing the National Commission:

> The commissioners typically reached conclusions by working inductively from specific examples to general principles. By moving from a common core of agreement outwards to its edges, they also showed just how extensive that core is. If the Commission had initially approached many of these issues as matter of principle, areas of pronounced disagreement might have emerged.[10]

Perhaps Capron had heard and been influenced by Toulmin's description of the National Commission by the time this account was written. Certainly his account of the President's Commission in this respect resembles that of Toulmin. To be consistent, Beauchamp and Childress would have to argue that Capron makes the same mistake as Toulmin, for no progress outward from a core of belief, to use Capron's image, would be possible without riding on some generalizing principles. To expand on this response, I would add that this does not mean that the commissioners did not each begin with certain principles, but rather that the principles were not so well defined that they presented a highly restricted range of choices. On the contrary, the Commission's consensus processes presented opportunities for the commissioners to learn more about the meanings of the principles they held as they went from case to case. It is because the moral principles held by the commissioners had a somewhat open texture that their group consensus could be enriched and expanded as they went. Had this not been the case, had their principles been highly defined and thereby restricted in application, their only alternative to an impasse would have been to negotiate in search of a compromise.

It is clear to me that, like principlism, casuistry does admit a role for justifying propositions, and that the difference lies in the epistemological status of the justifying propositions. My aim here, however, is not to enter the debate about casuistry but to illustrate a point about consensus and group processes. From the standpoint of group dynamics one can formulate a hypothesis that is compatible with both views about the National Commission's processes. This was a relatively well integrated and cooperative group that pursued its work in a spirit of mutual respect, while at the same time its members did not shrink from identifying and defending points of disagreement. When Jonsen and Toulmin suggest that the commissioners did not look closely at *why* they ultimately agreed (which Beauchamp and Childress interpret as a lack of certitude about theories, not principles), this can be taken as a sign that they were, on the whole, a harmonious working group.

Internal coherence is, however, no guarantee of external influence. As a part of the agency it was created to advise (the Department of Health, Education and Welfare), the National Commission was not always able to exert its authority. Thus, on several occasions, and contrary to law, the secretary either delayed his response to several regulations proposed by the Commission or ignored them entirely.[11] The consensus-building aspect of government commissions often requires more than crystallizing professional opinion; it may also entail galvanizing public opinion so as to put pressure on public officials to respect the commission's authority.

The President's Commission

For all the success of the National Commission in furthering the development of research ethics, no government ethics panel, whether in the United States or abroad, has been as influential as the President's Commission. Yet the scope of the President's Commission's work was far broader, and in some respects more subject to external political influences. In his retrospective analysis written shortly after the President's Commission completed its work in 1983, Capron, its executive director, drew contrasts with the National Commission. In particular Capron noted that the membership of the President's Commission rotated: "This meant that the Commission was more aware of the views of the incumbent administration and gave the President a greater stake in its work."[12] In less diplomatic terms, the

President's Commission was more exposed to shifting ideological currents than its predecessor. This structural feature proved to be of some political significance when President Carter was defeated and the conservative "Reagan revolution" came to Washington midway through the Commission's work.

Capron also calls attention to "the [President's Commission's] strong drive toward consensus . . . one that might have been predicted but was certainly not built in."[13] That the drive toward consensus was predictable is at least an understatement, given the obvious motivation for political leaders to assemble such a body. As I have already mentioned, one such motive is to build a broad base of popular support and intellectual justification for policy in an area that is a potential political mine field. Significantly, as Capron observes, only in the case of abortion was a subject considered unacceptably "divisive." In other words, in terms of the framework I have already developed, only abortion was so laden with fixed positions that the Commission's consensus processes would have been frayed by an effort to select a barely acceptable compromise, if one had even proved to be available.

That consensus need not have been the Commission's predominant operational model was noted in early analyses of its work by Robert A. Burt,[14] and by Alan J. Weisbard and John D. Arras.[15] One obvious alternative would be a "seminar" model, in which competing conceptualizations of crucial ideas such as that of the physician-patient relationship are exhaustively analyzed, with an implicit willingness to leave disagreements unresolved. While this might provide illumination and an occasion for public education, it would remain deeply unsatisfying to those who would wish such a body to achieve consensus. As a goal compromise would be somewhat more acceptable from a practical point of view, but it is a commonplace that compromise is intellectually frustrating and, in that sense, a last resort.

In general, however, Capron argues that the President's Commission went further than many might have thought possible in settling on some substantive moral positions. Agreement was reached, for example, not only that patients have a right to have life-sustaining treatment withheld, but that in some cases it may be permissible to withdraw treatment from, say, a permanently unconscious patient if another patient can be significantly benefited. In a peroration that reflects his sanguine view of the Commission's work, Capron in effect articulates the ideal for moral consensus processes in a pluralistic liberal democracy:

Rather than having harmful effects, the drive for consensus seems to have had a beneficial effect—it encouraged the commissioners to seek the common ground that best expresses the moral insights and values of Americans today, in light of our shared, albeit not uniform, religious and philosophical traditions.[16]

The structural arrangements of the President's Commission in at least one case subjected it to severe political constraints. Compared to its work on physician-patient relations, the determination of death, and genetic engineering, for example, the views expressed in the Commission's volume *Securing Access to Health Care*[17] have had little impact on the public debate. Indeed, the fate of *Securing Access* stands as a good example of the banality of superficial consensus. As Weisbard and Arras observed in a masterpiece of understatement:

When conservative Reagan appointees can agree with Carter-appointed liberals on a subject as highly politicized and divisive as health policy, one must wonder whether the substance of their agreement is likely to have any powerful implications for the formulation of health policy.[18]

Yet the appearance of consensus was achieved, but through what sort of process? In the discussion that follows I take advantage of the fact that much has been written about the process behind the President's Commission's report on access to health care, far more than is available concerning any other single report produced by the panel. This alone suggests that the process was in some way troubled. Thus, while there is surely much of a positive nature to learn about ethics commissions from the study of some of the other President's Commission reports, failure has a way of fixing the attention.

Ronald Bayer has assembled evidence showing that partisan politics intruded into the membership of the President's Commission at a critical juncture in its deliberations on access to health care. In early drafts of the report, Bayer claims, a rather explicit elaboration and defense of the idea of a right to health care was central. At around that time, however, some Carter administration appointees were cycling off the Commission and were replaced by Reagan administration appointees who made it clear to the Commission staff that they could not "buy into" that approach. Some staff members were so distressed, Bayer reports, that there was for a time danger of mass resignation and the creation of an independent staff report. The text that resulted from the strenuous intervention of chairman Abram and executive director Capron appealed in an eclectic manner to a strong societal obligation to provide a decent minimum level of health care. However cogent, this was a far less focused position than that originally staked out. Indeed, the rather strenuous arguments arrayed in favor of the strength of this obligation earlier in the text seem oddly detached from its cautious conclusion. In the final analysis, *Securing Access to Health Care* is really two documents. The body of the report represents staff consensus, while the conclusion is a compromise position worked out between the commissioners and the staff.[19]

In his review of the role of philosophers in the public policy process, Weisbard, a law professor who was one of the Commission's assistant directors, throws further light on the environment in which the Commission worked:

As a matter of conscious and explicit policy, reflecting the wishes and philosophies of the Commission's chairman and executive director, the Commission reached few conclusions, and made still fewer policy recommendations, that could not be endorsed unanimously, or nearly so, by the Commission members. This policy, coupled with formal and informal processes of consensus building with relevant professional communities and the Commission's openness to public comment and scrutiny, assured that the Commission's work would be broadly acceptable to diverse constituencies.[20]

Furthermore, in a footnote to their introduction to a symposium on the President's Commission, both Weisbard and Arras suggest a related reason for the gap between argument and conclusion in *Securing Access*: since the commissioners did not have the time or inclination to draft sections that concentrated on intellectual analysis, which were crafted exclusively by the staff, they tended to focus on conclusions. While the commissioners could require staff to redraft conclusions, they could not force them to come up with better arguments in support of these conclusions. The resulting "passive resistance" perhaps enabled the Commission's staff members to keep their consciences intact, but it detracted from the document's coherence.[21]

The point is not that politics should not play a role in small group deliberations, nor even that *partisan* politics can ever be wholly avoided, desirable as this might be. Rather, this example calls attention to the way an unfortunate conjunction of events can adversely affect a group's efforts to reach a consensus likely to have a significant influence. In this case unhappy timing brought in new group members in the middle of the drafting of a complex ethical, social, and financial statement. Politics, even of the partisan variety, does not necessarily preclude consensus formation so long as there is time for the factions to work out their modus operandi, and there are no pending issues that tend straightaway to stimulate defensive positions. The impression one has from the accounts I have mentioned is that the combination of factors in this case (new members, a partisan atmosphere, and a draft in midstream) was counterproductive. The Commission example also shows how badly needed was "a thoroughgoing analysis of the moral and institutional roles and responsibilities of Commission members and staff.[22]

It could be argued, of course, that no amount of time or energy would have enabled the commissioners to resolve their underlying philosophical differences on the status of health care in the marketplace. Yet on other vexed issues the dynamics of the President's Commission, even during this period, were of a quite different nature. The commissioners were able to agree on a critique of Reagan administration policy on the *Baby Doe* issue when that controversy erupted near the end of the Commission's tenure.[23] A different environment might at least have permitted the issues at stake to be clarified in a way that would have been useful for public debate rather than papered over.

But for our purposes the important lasting impression to take away from this particular Commission project is how powerful the drive for consensus was, in spite of the obstacles that became evident during the drafting of *Securing Access*. In his retrospective analysis Capron alludes carefully to the fact that eight commissioners were replaced in the final year of the Commission's work; thus, "the process of reasoning together in which the sitting commissioners had become adept had to be restarted with the newcomers."[24] Were one to draw any conclusions from this experience for national ethics commissions generally, it would be that continuity of membership and a concomitant insulation from partisan political shifts should be a part of the design, as was the case with the National Commission but not the President's Commission.

Governmental ethics commissions and political processes

In the foregoing formulation the salient term is "insulation," for while protection from relatively short-term ebbs and flows of partisan politics seems an unassailable desideratum of ethics commissions, it is not at all obvious that these panels should be altogether *isolated* from political currents. Were this the case they could not in principle meet one of their most important goals: to operate in a way that is relevant to the shared values of the society, addressing specific issues in light of the stable overlapping consensus. These issues can be addressed in two ways. An already emerging consensus can be articulated and reaffirmed, and authorities can be pressed to implement it (consensus-concluding); or an as-yet-unrealized consensus can be framed, tested, revised, and promoted to the general public as well as to particular stakeholders, such as professional organizations (consensus-developing).

For example, Capron argues that the President's Commission played the consensus-concluding role with respect to recommendations on research regulation that had lain dormant since the work of the National Commission, and that it played the consensus-developing role with regard to physician-patient relations in medical decision making. In his own analysis Capron adds a third function, that of a "lightning rod" for an issue of public concern that the conventional political process is not well designed to manage. His example is the President's Commission's report on fetal research.[25] Although this is a quibble, it seems to me that the difference between the second and third examples is one of degree rather than of kind, and that both are instances in which unresolved ethical issues carry varying degrees of political freight. From Capron's point of view the distinction between the cases is understandable, since he believes the effort on medical decision making to have succeeded and that on fetal research to have largely failed. But the outcome does not distinguish the intended commission function, which was, in my view, one of consensus development in both cases.

The interests of political leaders and society dovetail in both goals of national ethics commissions. In the consensus-conclusion process political leaders and the polity are well served when an implicit but previously unrecognized consensus can finally be established as part of social policy. In the process of consensus development both elected officials and the society may avoid a wasteful conflict in which morality and politics become hopelessly confused and principles rigidly defined: the classic example is, again, abortion.

There are, moreover, few risks involved in forming a panel to deal with a morally problematic area. In spite of the possibility that a delayed response will aggravate the situation or the appearance of timidity by public officials, the stated purpose of guarding or building consensus is in itself hard to criticize. Weisbard puts the point concisely in his realistic assessment of reasons for the President's Commission's apparent success:

[O]ne should not overlook the understandable readiness of officials in all branches of government—judicial as well as legislative and executive—to deflect *personal* responsibility (and potential political vulnerability) for decisions on highly charged and value-laden questions by explicitly adopting the moderate and mainstream recommendations of a seemingly expert, non-partisan and objective "ethics commission." Indeed, political actors may appear statesmanlike in doing so.[26]

In 1993 the U.S. Congress's Office of Technology Assessment (OTA) published a report called *Biomedical Ethics in U.S. Public Policy*. Working with an advisory panel of bioethicists, the OTA summarized the historic experience of government ethics commissions with an eye toward the question whether another one should soon be established, and if so, how it should be organized. Concerning the latter point, the report offered a general conclusion:

Successful commissions were relatively free of political interference, had flexibility in addressing issues, were open in their process and dissemination of findings, and were comprised of a diverse group of individuals who were generally free of ideology and had wide ranging experience.[27]

This conclusion on the whole squares with the observations made by Weisbard and others. Other sensible propositions that are also expressed in the OTA report essentially follow from this one. For example, the report emphasized that commissions should not be burdened with a mandate that includes issues likely to be a priori divisive, such as abortion, and that suitable funding would enable a staff of professional bioethicists to assess particular points of view in a detached manner. It also urged that the structure of a commission should follow from its scope and issues, since a standing body would be suitable for some purposes, a term-limited body for others.

Of particular interest is the report's assumptions concerning the role of commissions with regard to consensus in public policy on bioethical issues. On the whole, the report encourages Congress to appoint another bioethics commission, for, as it pointedly notes,

[f]or nearly 4 years—the longest period of time since bioethics burgeoned as a discipline—the Federal Government has been without a formal forum that addresses bioethical issues. In fact, a full operational body has not existed in over a decade.[28]

At several points in the report consensus and "consensus building" are mentioned in ways that suggest that this is an important reason for establishing another commission, yet the authors seem decidedly ambivalent about the precise significance of commission consensus. For example, it is asserted that "commissions can clarify issues and offer useful critiques of public policy, but they lack the moral and political authority to decide what ought to be done." But a few lines later we read that commissions "can provide a broadly accepted basis for understanding the issues and propose particular policies to cover most situations."[29] Of course, the idea that an ethics panel can help in "understanding the issues" and proposing policies is about as minimal as one can get, nor are these functions that can be served only by ethics commissions. More important, if the language of "a broadly accepted basis" is not a surrogate for the word *consensus*, then one might at least wonder how commmissions' recommendations can be broadly accepted if "they lack the moral and political authority to decide what ought to be done"!

My purpose here is not to be pedantic. The OTA report is in other respects careful and therefore typical of what we have come to expect from this agency. Thus it is all the more striking that important questions about the authority of consensus slide by. It is clear from some of the remarks and citations in the report that these questions did occur to the authors. The fact that they were not articulated as clearly as they might have been, and that ambiguities of the kind I have described resulted, can perhaps be explained by the tension between the intellectual interests and qualifications of the OTA staff and the politically attractive nature of ethics commissions in a diverse and democratic society, a tension reminiscent of the situation of ethics commissions themselves. The OTA's goal was, after all, to provide the Congress with an account of ethics commissions. As I have argued, the essential attraction of ethics commissions for legislators and others concerned with the making of public policy has in practice been a political one. In the next section I discuss one of the more important of these questions about consensus in a liberal polity.

Ethics commissions and the limits of liberalism

The essential criticism of ethics commissions is stated in the clearest possible terms by Jay Katz in his commentary on the President's Commission: "Inevitable obfuscations emerge whenever commissions strive for a consensus report about complex moral dilemmas." Katz reasons that any consensus about "a fundamental reorientation in ethical practices" tends to obscure the problems of implementation; and perhaps more seriously, "morality . . . requires the presentation of disparate views."[30] Here Katz makes a critical point, for consensus does render dissent less obvious. Indeed if it did not, there would hardly be any reason to pursue broad agreement. But surely an important element of a democratic society is the persistence of dissent, of a loyal opposition. As the questions become more fundamental and more difficult, as in the case of the issues considered by national ethics commissions, the importance of the opposition increases. In the same law review volume in which Katz's article appears, Robert A. Burt makes a similar point, that in striving for consensus on gut-wrenching issues such as the termination of treatment for seriously ill infants, the Commission attempted to be reassuring. The net result was that certain conceptions of parental duties toward children, for example, inevitably suffer as others are endorsed.[31]

To these views can be opposed that of Morris Abram, the chairman of the President's Commission, and Susan Wolf, who argue that "consensus among commission members [is] essential" because a commission has only the power of persuasion.

Unlike a court or legislature, which is structured to have effect as long as a majority agrees, a commission requires agreement that is as close to unanimity as possible, to have any effect at all.[32]

Abram and Wolf stress the commission's role as a source of persuasive argument, appealing presumably to reason rather than emotion and not as a source of legal fiat. In enlarging on this premise Katz's view would have more force if a commission were a legislative body, but in fact it is one voice (however distinguished) among others. Therefore it is a party to the debate rather than the rubric under which the entire social conversation takes place.

On one point, however, Katz's position is unassailable: in any set of recommendations reached by consensus the public should have access to information about the deliberative process. "Arriving at an acceptable consensus document must have been laden with agonizing choices," Katz observes, "which discretion precluded airing."[33] The same may be said about any consensus process, whether in ethics commissions or committees, that those who are directly affected by the results deserve to know the woof and warp of the deliberations. This condition appears to require more than the usual quasi-academic rehearsal of the most persuasive arguments on each side; rather, it calls for an airing of the options not not chosen, along with the practical as well as the theoretical considerations that ultimately weighed against their selection.

Thus, ethics commissions do not only serve disinterested intellectual goals; their primary function is to preserve social peace. This does not give them license to produce intellectually shoddy work. But it must be recognized in all candor that, in a democratic society, ethics commissions are at least a mechanism for reducing conflict about moral questions, and perhaps even for accomplishing a social consensus. At a minimum it must be conceded that moral philosophy does not present moral theories that deliver unambiguous answers to public policy questions. As Will Kymlicka notes: "Utilitarians disagree amongst themselves about the acceptability of surrogacy, or the status of the embryo, as do proponents of all the other theories."[34] The evaluation of an ethics commission's performance requires a framework that marries moral and political philosophy. Liberal political philosophy is a promising framework, but it is only a beginning.

As Kymlicka goes on to argue, just as moral philosophers disagree, so also must the diversity of viewpoints within the society be recognized in some way by the commission. But the recognition of diversity is not, as we have seen, the mark of success that ethics commissions have tended to set for themselves. Instead they have sought to articulate and, if possible, extend societal consensus. In a liberal and pluralistic society the justifiability of a commission's conclusions depends, at a minimum, on whether they can be sanctioned by principles that are objects of a broad consensus. These conclusions also demand attention to the informal political, sociological, and psychological factors that condition them. However impressive the credentials of their participants and effectual their conclusions, the study of ethics commissions reminds us that consensus is not desirable in itself and at any price. In particular, it also indicates the limitations of the political rationale for the authority of moral consensus.

Notes

1. F. Mullan et al., "The Town Meeting for Technology: The Maturation of Consensus Conferences," *Journal of the American Medical Association* 254, 8 (1985): 1068–72.
2. Ibid., p. 1068.
3. Veatch, "Consensus of Expertise."
4. This summary is based on LeRoy Walters, "Commissions and Bioethics," *Journal of Medicine and Philosophy* 14, 4 (1989): 363–68.
5. National Commission for the Protection of Human Subjects of Biomedical and Behavioral Research, "Belmont Report: Ethical Principles and Guidelines for the Protection of Human Subjects of Research," *Federal Register* 44, 76 (1979): 23, 192–97.
6. See George Annas and Michael Grodin, *The Nazi Doctors' Trial and the Nuremberg Code* (New York: Oxford University Press, 1993).
7. Beauchamp and Childress, *Principles of Biomedical Ethics*, 4th ed.
8. Jonsen and Toulmin, *Abuse of Casuistry*.
9. Beauchamp and Childress, *Principles of Biomedical Ethics*, 4th ed., pp. 92–99.
10. Alexander Morgan Capron, "Looking Back at the President's Commission," *Hastings Center Report* 13, 5 (1983): 8.
11. Joseph Palca, "The Fifth Commission," *Hastings Center Report* 23, 4 (1993): 5.
12. Capron, "Looking Back at the President's Commission," p. 7.
13. Ibid., p. 8.
14. Robert A. Burt, "The Ideal of Community in the Work of the President's Commission," *Cardozo Law Review* 6, 2 (1984): 267-86.
15. Alan J. Weisbard and John D. Arras, "Commissioning Morality: An Introduction to the Symposium," *Cardozo Law Review* 6, 2 (1984): 223–41.
16. Capron, "Looking Back at the President's Commission," p. 8.
17. President's Commission for the Study of Ethical Problems in Medicine and Biomedical and Behavioral Research, *Securing Access to Health Care: The Ethical Implications of Differences in the Availability of Health Services* (Washington, D.C.: U.S. Government Printing Office, 1983).
18. Weisbard and Arras, "Commissioning Morality," p. 238, n. 66.
19. Ronald Bayer, "Ethics, Politics, and Access to Health Care: A Critical Analysis of the President's Commission for the Study of Ethical Problems in Medicine and Biomedical and Behavioral Research," *Cardozo Law Review* 6, 2 (1984): 303–20.
20. Alan J. Weisbard, "The Role of Philosophers in the Public Policy Process: A View from the President's Commission," *Ethics* 97, 3 (1987): 777.
21. Weisbard and Arras, "Commissioning Morality," p. 233, n. 45.
22. Ibid., p. 233, n. 45.

23. Weisbard, "The Role of Philosophers in the Public Policy Process," p. 777, n. 3.
24. Capron, "Looking Back at the President's Commission," p. 8.
25. Ibid., p. 9.
26. Weisbard, "The Role of Philosophers in the Public Policy Process," p. 778.
27. U.S. Congress, Office of Technology Assessment, *Biomedical Ethics in U.S. Public Policy*, p. 18.
28. Ibid., p. 25.
29. Ibid., p. 27.
30. Jay Katz, "Limping Is No Sin: Reflections on *Making Health Care Decisions*," *Cardozo Law Review* 6, 2 (1984): 246.
31. Burt, "The Ideal of Community in the Work of the President's Commission."
32. Morris Abram and Susan Wolf, "Public Involvement in Medical Ethics: A Model for Government Action," *New England Journal of Medicine* 310, 10 (1984): 629.
33. Katz, "Limping Is No Sin," p. 247.
34. Will Kymlicka, "Moral Philosophy and Public Policy," *Bioethics* 7, 1 (1991): 7.

6

Healthcare Ethics Committees

The healthcare ethics committee movement

Whereas ethics commissions focus on policies that are to apply across institutions, ethics committees are creatures of particular institutions. Their legal and bureaucratic authority is established by administration or by a medical staff organization, but their ultimate responsibility is supposed to be to the patients. They are expected to be respectful of legal constraints, disciplinary integrity, and institutional protocols but also to be critical of them and, if necessary, to appeal to higher sources of guidance, such as philosophical reflection.

Perhaps the only element of the modern ethics committee's mission that is taken as mandatory is the protection of patients' personal autonomy. So long as committees hew closely to this line, their activities appear to be strongly validated in a liberal society. Yet in particular cases and in pluralistic environments it is not always easy to tell how to satisfy this standard. Despite this limitation in detail, the idea of using facility-based committees to interpret the implications of an overlapping consensus has immense political appeal, especially in the United States.

Later in this chapter I review the history of the ethics committee movement in the United States, including the reasons for the periodic spurts in the number of committees. For now, it is enough to establish the fact of considerable growth. Working within a rather narrow definition, the President's Commission reported in 1982 that ethics committees could be found in only 1 percent of hospitals sampled.[1] In 1983, 26 percent of respondents to an American Hospital Association (AHA) study reported having ethics committees.[2] Two years later another AHA study found that number had risen to 60 percent.[3] That this trend has continued in all sorts of health care institutions is evidenced by a 1988 survey of army hospitals, which found that 76 percent had ethics committees.[4] Although there is no question that there has been considerable growth in the number of such bodies, at least two caveats are in order: first, the surveys did not all define ethics committee in the same way; and second, even those ethics committees that were accurately reported within the survey definition varied greatly in the extent to which they actually functioned.

It is a commonplace in the literature that the definition of an ethics committee is elusive. Recognizing that the proliferation of ethics committees as a part of the health care system has outrun our understanding of them, this book engages primarily theoretical problems that are stimulated by the idea of an ethics committee. This idea can be expressed in many ways, but roughly I take it to be this: when health care decision making engages value questions about which society is evidently unsettled, then it is often advisable to seek the deliberative assistance of a group which, though diverse, includes individuals who are familiar with the social institutions that are likely to be relevant, thus representing medicine, nursing, law, hospital administration, social work, philosophy, religion, and so forth.

Two comments concerning the actual implementation of this idea bear further elaboration. First, one can validly raise the question whether the term *ethics committee* is a misnomer (as one can for ethics commissions) and argue that what really goes on in most such bodies is another form of administrative or quasi-legal review. For the time being I will assume that at least some of what goes on in a typical ethics committee's deliberations is readily identifiable as within the scope of ethics, and that this is central to its activities. Second, no one who has experienced more than one nominal ethics committee can fail to be impressed by the enormous variation in process and quality. The theoretical considerations addressed in this book relate to those more settled committees that are generally regarded as successful by those who have availed themselves of their services. How to construe this apparent success is of course one of my basic concerns.

One can distinguish three different sorts of institutional committees in the American health care system which have more or less explicitly ethical charges concerning human beings: institutional review boards (IRBs), which, among other things, monitor the use of human subjects in research; infant care review committees (ICRCs), which consider questions about the care of newborns, especially in neonatal intensive care units; and healthcare ethics committees (HECs), which are mainly concerned with ethical questions involving adults and older children. IRBs, which have more of a policing function than ICRCs and HECs, are responsible for ensuring that the statutory requirements of specific federal legislation are respected. In this legal capacity clear-cut majority views become more important than in ICRCs, which are responsive mainly to rather general federal requirements of states to investigate complaints of nontreatment of a handicapped infant. Since HECs are not usually associated with government regulation of health care, they have still more flexibility than ICRCs to determine their own functions, including the manner in which their collective views are to be determined. The term *ethics committee* is used in this book to refer to HECs primarily and ICRCs secondarily; although a number of nursing ethics committees have also been established, it is not clear that most of them engage in the case and policy review characteristic of general institutional or departmental ethics committees. Of course, much of what is said in this book about the philosophy and sociology of consensus in small groups applies to IRBs as well, and generally to those bureaucratic creatures called committees.

The freedom of ethics committees to function according to their own design may change as governmental and accrediting bodies require or encourage health care institutions to create them. The state of Maryland mandates them of all health care institutions, though as yet without requirements for composition and procedures. New York State's Task Force on Life and the Law has proposed mandating the participation of "bioethics review committees" in making certain decisions on behalf of patients lacking advance directives or appointed surrogates.[5] And the Joint Commission for the Accreditation of Healthcare Organizations now requires its members to establish procedures for "ethics review," which could presumably be satisfied by an HEC or an ethics consultant or some combination of the two.[6]

In a formal sense, the vast majority of institutional ethics committees regard their role as "advisory"; rarely are their findings mandatory for the parties to a controversy. Regardless of the status of an ethics committee's recommendations, whether advisory or mandatory, the committee's function is to arrive at some conclusion. Even if a committee demurs from giving advice in a certain case, that is still a decision that the group has reached, albeit a negative and nonsubstantive one. Furthermore, the distinction between advisory and mandatory opinions is often more apparent than real. For example, under certain political conditions the supposedly advisory nature of an ethics committee's views could be difficult for the principals to ignore, as when the chair of the hospital board or the chief of the medical staff is also chair of the ethics committee.

In the context of case review and policy advisement, there is probably an overemphasis in the literature on the identification of a single best alternative as the result of an ethics committee's deliberations. Instead, a well-functioning and mature committee may prefer to identify a range of morally acceptable alternatives with regard, for example, to appropriate management of the terminally ill patient. Therefore, the idea of consensus does not only apply when a single best alternative is being sought. To the contrary, consensus processes surely must also be operative when a morally acceptable *range* of management alternatives is being identified.

Whether or not ethics committees operate according to consensus rather than, say, a majority vote is partly an empirical question. Evidence from survey data indicates that most ethics committee members characterize their approach in terms of developing a consensus. In the most comprehensive comparative study of ethics committees, from 75 to 92 percent of committee members reported that decisions are made by means of consensus, with most of the remainder reporting that votes are taken.[7] Of course, what precisely is meant by consensus in this context is not entirely clear. There are at least three possible meanings: (1) the positive view of all or virtually all individual committee members; (2) the product of an effort to accommodate the views of all or virtually all committee members (a sort of coordination problem); or (3) an attempt by the committee members to replicate what all or virtually all of them think would be morally acceptable to the relevant larger community. This ambiguity raises interesting questions about the self-perception of ethics committee members as they engage in their activities.

Ethics committees as committees

In the trivial sense that they represent bureaucratic lines of authority and control, all committees are political entities. It is therefore no wonder that ethics committees have adopted the standard of consensus, for consensus, like autonomy, is a political concept that has been imported into ethical territory. But unlike the concept of autonomy, consensus has not yet undergone systematic and intense scrutiny in medical ethics. To this end much can be learned from social scientists. As I mentioned in the first chapter, unlike philosophers, who seem often to assume that consensus is an active process, sociologists distinguish between consensus by "head count" and by acquiescence.[8] The study of patterns of small group interaction can also be informative, as the next chapter will illustrate. Whether the committee's conclusions are optional or mandatory, and whether it reviews or makes policy, we need to know what moral weight to ascribe to committee positions. This requires further theoretical and empirical examination of the actual operation of consensus.

Some contend that, owing to their inherently political nature, committees can never be more than reflections of established powers, poor sites for resolving an institution's moral quandaries.[9] Certainly a committee system can easily lead to abuse, since members may be held in thrall by the authorities who have appointed them. I am not prepared to concede that committees are necessarily corrupt for purposes of ethical consultation, though their nature warrants caution.[10]

It might be argued that there is no interesting difference between an ethics committee and any other bureaucratic entity in a complex social structure such as a hospital. What distinguishes it is not its multidisciplinary membership, its procedures, or its political or legal functions, all of which might be similar to those of other committees. Rather, according to this view, the only difference is that the content of its issues is, or is supposed to be, specifically ethical in nature. These issues merely fall into one category of medical practice and administration, a category for which a certain sort of committee is established. In the hospital management scheme the ethics committee fills a niche similar to those filled by many others. Thus, one could argue there is no reason at all why consensus should not close discussion in ethics committees, as it may for any committee operating in and for the institution. On this view, a simple majority would be definitive were it not for the odd notion that ethics should not be a matter of majority rule (though hardheaded social observers tell us that it often is).

Moreover, the actual work of many of these bodies does not always consist in helping resolve ethical disputes as a moral philosopher or theologian would understand that concept. Indeed, addressing communication problems, searching for additional facts, or uncovering medicolegal misconceptions are among the activities typical of ethics committees. The diverse and often contentious activity of ethics committees has been described elsewhere.[11] Even when genuinely ethical issues arise, often the committee' task is to identify the authoritative literature and apply its conclusions. Paradoxically, ethics committees do not always, or even usually, worry over ethical dilemmas. This state of affairs is less surprising when it is recalled that the term was popularized through the *Quinlan* decision by a court that was actually talking about prognosis committees.[12]

Yet there are at least two good reasons to worry about the moral authority of consensus in ethics committees. First, some of these committees do find themselves asked to comment on hard cases or institutional policy options involving conflicts of moral values. Second, merely because of their name ethics committees will often be seen as lending a special kind of authority to their advice even if the content of the advice does not concern a moral dilemma strictly speaking.

The potential for the ethics committee to be perceived as a unique authority in a hospital is apparent in another way. Unlike other committees in an institution, in principle the ethics committee may reasonably withdraw from a case without being viewed as having abdicated its responsibilities (unless, as is the case in several states, ethics committees have statutory authority).[13] If no solution acceptable to all parties seems available, the committee may take the position that it would be inappropriate for it to force a particular point of view in a morally vague area, for to do so would leave the impression that it is reasonable to force a single committee's ethical consensus on everyone else.

An ethics committee's withdrawal from a controversy would effectively leave the problem to an administrative or legal remedy. In fact, most committees stress an "advisory" rather than a "decision-making" capacity, regarding their functions as mediation and the improvement of communication. As if to emphasize this, some committees do not even call themselves committees but use some less suggestive title such as "group" or "forum." This characteristic also partly distinguishes the present-day ethics committee from other bodies in the history of medical decision making which have performed tasks with ethical implications, including, for example, kidney dialysis allocation committees. It would have been far more difficult for those other entities to withdraw from a controversy and retain their status in the institution.

Toward a history of ethics committees

The recent growth of consensus-based ethics committees in health care decision making obscures the resistance with which they were met by physicians and clinical investigators. Even panels composed entirely of doctors and medical scientists have been regarded as intrusions on the judgment and prerogatives of the individual practitioner, a vestige of the oft-cited paternalism of traditional medicine. It is interesting to note, for example, the view expressed in 1964 by a report to the director of the National Institutes of Health. This document, commonly referred to as the Livingston Report, was a response to the revelation that elderly patients at the Brooklyn Jewish Chronic Disease Hospital had been injected with live cancer cells without their knowledge or consent. The Livingston Report was a precursor to the requirement by the Public Health Service of prior review for all research projects involving human subjects. Despite the scandal that motivated the Livingston Report and the committee review system that finally emerged, its author expressed the opinion that

Group consensus as to what should be permitted, what could be done, and what would be of value may be far less reasonable than the considered view of a single fully qualified investigator.[14]

Indeed, the history of ethics committees can be regarded as a gradual but inexorable reduction of the discretion of the individual physician.

There have been to date four important periods in the history of ethics committees. First came the prehistory of ethics committees, represented by various examples of moral decision making by small groups in contexts that have more or less to do with medicine and health care. Second, the early history of ethics committees, dating from about the time of the *Quinlan* decision, evidenced a confusion about their function. Third, the more recent history of ethics committees, including a President's Commission report and the federal "Baby Doe" rules, saw an increase both in their popularity and in confusion about their goals. At the end of the chapter I will discuss the fourth period, which the movement is now entering, a period in which the committees are being viewed as potential regulatory devices; this development involves federal and state legislation, institutional credentialing, and the bureaucratization of the ethics committee movement.

As I shall attempt to show, there can be no doubt about one important reason for the historic interest in committees for ethical review, and for their recent surge in popularity: they provide a politically attractive way for moral controversies to be procedurally accommodated. A reconstruction of the increasing acceptability of ethics committees since *Quinlan* is a particularly vivid demonstration, as we shall see. To me this contingent fact does not damn the idea of an ethics committee (though it will in the eyes of some), but it does reinforce the notion that the quest for moral consensus is of a piece with broadly acceptable political arrangements, especially in a liberal democracy.

The prehistory of the contemporary ethics committee is surprisingly rich, for the idea of authorizing small groups to make ethical decisions or give recommendations concerning medical treatment is not a new one. This evolving line includes a number of different species, among them sterilization committees for the "feeble-minded," abortion review committees, kidney dialysis selection committees, and institutional review boards. On the basis of this list alone one can guess that the record of these precursors to modern ethics committees is not necessarily one that the proponents of HECs should want to celebrate. I shall briefly review each of these predecessors, paying special attention to the role that moral consensus played in the concept and operation of these committees.

Sterilization Committees

Nonvoluntary or involuntary sterilization for eugenic purposes was a significant social movement in the United States during roughly the first third of the twentieth century, one that was led by numerous respectable intellectuals and health care theorists. The sterilization of those labeled idiots, morons, or mental defectives (sometimes including criminals) is an example of negative eugenics, as selective breeding for the creation of superior individuals is called positive eugenics. The Supreme Court decision in *Buck v. Bell* (1927)[15] gave judicial support to negative eugenics policies that were by then embodied in the laws of most states. The eugenics movement collapsed with revelations of Nazi enthusiasm for eugenics (though there are those who claim its spirit persists in modern genetic testing practices). In addition to its political unpalatability, by midcentury the conceptual shortcomings of eugenics had become increasingly apparent, for few mental disabilities are heritable, nor can genius be created by selective mating.

Committees played a significant role in the sterilization system in the United States. Although these committees were normally composed of physicians, J. H. Landman, writing in 1932, was rather critical of the assumption that M.D.'s were well qualified for this job.[16] Physicians likely to be involved were usually expert in psychology and psychiatry but lacked training in heredity and biology. Several states required other professionals to sit on these committees, such as neurologists or sociologists. In retrospect, given the intellectual confusions on which eugenic sterilization was based, none of these professions can be said to have performed terribly well through its committee representatives.

Only a few statutes still permit sterilization of institutionalized individuals based on the findings of an expert panel without any judicial review and even in those cases they are unlikely to be acted upon.[17] What has changed since the heyday of sterilization is not only the way the idea of due process is applied but also the *justification* for sterilization. Formerly sterilization was performed largely for eugenic purposes, to benefit society at large. The "patient" might also benefit by being relieved of the burden of sexual impulse, but this was a secondary consideration. By contrast, *therapeutic* sterilization is supposed to be performed for the benefit of the patient and no one else, and the burden of proof is decidedly on the party urging that the procedure would be a benefit to the individual.

Revealing in the history of sterilization committees is the uncertainty about suitability for membership on the committees. In his 1932 commentary Landman observed that physicians were often no better schooled in the relevant subjects than liberal arts college graduates, and that many committee members were appointed by institutional superintendents, who were themselves often political appointees rather than psychologists or psychiatrists.[18] Thus, both the knowledge base of the committee members and their personal suitability for the job were called into question. These criticisms (the lack of relevant expertise and presence of a political agenda) are strikingly reminiscent of criticisms that have been leveled at modern ethics committees.

Abortion Review Committees

By 1970 abortion law reforms had been passed by a dozen states in response to charges by post–World War II abortion rights activists that many women who wanted abortions did not have access to them. These statutes required some review authority, including either a certain number of consultants, a therapeutic abortion board, or a hospital review authority. The last could consist of from one to three members, and the required approval varied from majority to unanimity. Panels could easily be manipulated, such as by placing a firmly antiabortion physician on a review board that required unanimity.[19]

In spite of these limitations, committees were the most popular method for determining who would be able to have a therapeutic abortion, beginning with the committee founded in 1945 by Alan Guttmacher. Defenders of the committees argued that they would deter "indiscriminate" abortion, act in the patient's best interests, provide physicians with a medicolegal safeguard, and serve as a repository of data about interrupted pregnancies. Opponents of abortion review committees charged that they were a smokescreen for physicians who wished to protect themselves from public criticism by hiding behind what consensus theory understands as the irresponsibility of the group. Others noted that any particular committee could be constituted so that abortions were virtually banned or virtually unrestricted. Still others voiced the hope that lawyers and legislators would eventually "turn the problem back to doctors where it belongs."[20] In their 1973 history of abortion, published just before the revolution of *Roe v. Wade*, Betty Sarvis and Hyman Rodman offered by way of laconic comment what was perhaps the most that could be said on behalf of these review panels:

[A]bortion committees clearly serve a purpose for hospitals and physicians in a situation where little consensus can be achieved and where the law leaves the decision in medical hands.[21]

In fact, however, considerable consensus seems to have been achieved within the committees themselves—even if not in society at large—or at least no deep differences in points of view among the members were reported. This could be attributed either to professional etiquette in not publicizing such differences, or to a deliberate selection of members with roughly similar views on the matter. Finally, there were significant differences among the committees in the proportion of rejected requests for abortions, ranging from 25 percent at one California hospital to 60 percent at another.[22]

Kidney Dialysis Selection Committees

Perhaps the single best known review committee in the history of biomedical ethics was the group that made allocation decisions for chronic hemodialysis at Swedish Hospital in Seattle, Washington, during the early 1960s. Immortalized by Shana Alexander in a much-reprinted *Life* magazine story, the committee was composed wholly of lay persons, upright citizens and members of the community. The salient point of Alexander's story was the impression that the members had little difficulty reaching life-or-death decisions based on their shared middle-class values. Operating in a determinedly utilitarian milieu, they found the middle-aged male bank officer with a wife and three children to be a superior candidate, in comparison to the older unemployed "former" alcoholic with no dependents. To their credit, the members of the "God committee" expressed discomfort with their own processes.[23]

Physicians expressed the usual reservations about lay intrusions in the doctor-patient relationship, but by this time it was widely appreciated that the decisions involved went beyond individual professional-client relationships. Most of the academic discussion of selection for life-saving dialysis has focused on the use of criteria of social worth and to a lesser extent on the problem of representing other than middle-class values on such bodies. The place of consensus in this episode, however, raises questions that are at least as fundamental as these. Consider that the committee members were operating on two levels of consensus. The first was the level of the values that they brought with them into the room, values that *in this case* seemed to validate certain operating principles, albeit largely tacit and unarticulated principles. This can be construed as an appeal to the society's overlapping consensus. The second was the level of values that they manifested when they made their specific decisions. When there were disagreements about these particular cases, they were forced to go back to their largely unexpressed background theory and see if they could find a reason for the disagreement that might also provide a shared basis for resolving it. Even for those of us whose philosophy of science is a bit rusty, this iterative process is highly reminiscent of the cycle from theory to anomalous observation and back to theory again.

A de facto set of background values or principles is a common characteristic of all the kinds of committees covered in our history so far, even if not articulated as such, and apart from the cogency of the idea of an overlapping consensus. This value set may come from a common professional or intellectual background, or from a shared cultural sensibility, or both. As we move into the period of government and other official forms of ethics regulation, we find that the guiding principles that are presumed to be objects of committee consensus a priori, before review of specific cases, become explicit.

Institutional Review Boards

By the mid-1970s federal rules were in place requiring the systematic review of government-sponsored research involving human subjects. Since the early 1960s a number of institutions had created institutional review boards on their own initiative. Federal legislation mandated and regularized IRBs, including a requirement for diversity of membership: that is, no IRB could be entirely all male or all female, and (so far as was reasonable, given the institution's location) a variety of racial and cultural groups had to be represented. In addition, the rules specified that there must be at least one "nonscientific" member, as well as individuals representing several disciplines.[24]

From the movement toward IRBs in general, one can infer an appreciation at the federal level that decisions concerning human beings in research are not purely scientific matters, but also they involve the consideration of moral values. In its landmark "Belmont Report," discussed in the preceding chapter, the National Commission had already spelled out the relevant ethical principles as respect for persons, beneficence, and justice. The membership requirements can be construed as an effort to implement the first principle. The Department of Health and Human Services, in setting forth the requirements, stated that "diverse membership is important and should enhance the IRB's credibility as well as insure a sensitivity to the concerns of both investigators and human research subjects."[25]

But it would be naive to conclude that ensuring recognition of community values by a diverse IRB membership has as an unalloyed purpose preserving the principle of respect for persons. To put it somewhat crudely, the use of human subjects creates potentially serious political problems for the research enterprise, especially in communities made up of many vulnerable people; the Tuskegee experience remains among the most pertinent cases in point. While respect for

persons and avoidance of adverse publicity may happen to be compatible, in practical terms it is also true that any threat of the latter helps to ensure that the former
is taken seriously. A Food and Drug Administration (FDA) communication about
IRBs in locations other than those where research is to be held states that "[t]he
nonlocal IRB must be knowledgeable about the community from which the subjects are drawn to ensure that their rights will be protected and that the consent
process is appropriate for the subject population involved."[26] "Rights" are not
usually thought to vary greatly from one locality to another (except, of course,
for legal rights), and the FDA has never officially adopted a philosophy of moral
relativism. Thus, I am inclined to read such statements more in terms of official
concern about public reaction than about upholding the ethical principle of respect for persons.

In any case, the IRB movement is distinctive in that it led to statutory requirements for an ethics committee review of processes that would formerly have been
considered strictly matters of professional competence. Also significant is the fact
that specific standards of judgment are imposed on all such bodies in the form of
the three ethical principles. Although diversity of membership may indeed help
implement respect for persons, it does not resolve in advance the problem of determining what counts as the satisfaction of this principle, or of beneficence, or
justice. Those decisions are, once again, largely matters of group consensus.

Quinlan: appearance and reality

The New Jersey Supreme Court's 1976 decision in the case of Karen Anne Quinlan
is recognized mainly for certifying the legal right of formerly competent patients
to refuse treatment. But this decision also qualifies as much as any other single
event as the beginning of the modern healthcare ethics committee. In the course
of recommending that hospitals establish ethics committees in such cases as a way
of avoiding time-consuming and costly litigation, the Justices cited a law review
article written by a pediatrician, Dr. Karen Teel, who stated:

[M]any hospitals have established an Ethics Committee composed of physicians, social
workers, attorneys, and theologians . . . which serves to review individual circumstances
of ethical dilemmas and which has provided much in the way of assistance and safeguards
for patients and their medical caretakers.[27]

In addition to its exaggeration of the prevalence of ethics committees in the early
1970s, a further and far more significant peculiarity of this view is that, as
the *Quinlan* text indicates, the Court's concept of an ethics committee turns out
not to square with Dr. Teel's. The Court's committee was to consist wholly of
physicians, and would in this case have been consulted for its agreement "that
there is no reasonable possibility of Karen's ever emerging from her present
comatose condition to a cognitive sapient state." With this sort of mechanism, said
the Court, the request from parents, guardians, and physicians that Karen be re-

moved from life-sustaining treatment would be immune from civil or criminal liability. Thus the court was describing not an ethics committee in the pure sense but a prognosis committee to review the attending physician's assessment of the patient's condition.[28]

Setting aside the problem of the composition of the committee envisioned by the *Quinlan* Court, one could argue that there was an unstated premise in the Justices' presentation, namely, that settlement of the prognosis issue was an essential condition for a sound ethical determination. While this is indisputable, there remains the strictly ethical problem that some moral principles would appear to prohibit the removal of life-sustaining therapy even in the event of a dismal prognosis. There are two related ironies in this ambiguous milestone in the history of ethics committees. The first is obviously that the influence of the *Quinlan* decision in creating an impetus for the establishment of ethics committees is somewhat misplaced. The second is that, although the Justices did not quite get it right, some of the business of at least some ethics committees probably does draw them into clinical determinations as well as strictly ethical dilemmas.

A further irony is that *Quinlan* lent credence to the notion that ethics committees could legally immunize hospitals and physicians, or at least greatly reduce the chance of successful litigation against them. Surely this is one of the less exalted but more prominent reasons why so many institutions and professionals have taken an interest in them, leading in large measure to the "growth industry" in HECs. But again, the multidisciplinary panel envisioned by Teel is one thing, the all-physician review group described by the *Quinlan* court another. Indeed, a line of cases from the late 1970s to the early 1980s gives a contradictory impression. In *Saikewicz* (1977)[29] the Court strongly discouraged committees as substitutes for the courts; in *Storar* (1981)[30] only the patient was allowed to refuse treatment; and in *Colyer* the Court advocated a medical "prognosis board," but not an ethics committee with nonphysicians as members.[31]

These results in the aftermath of *Quinlan* suggest that the legal system was by no means prepared to embrace the ethics committee concept. Hence, early confidence among some about the protection afforded hospitals and professionals may not have been well founded. In the years since these decisions, however, the situation has arguably changed. If that is so, and if these committees are now likely to enjoy greater legal acceptance, this is not because of an independent change in the way judges view them so much as it is due to legislative and regulatory changes that the courts themselves must recognize.

Before I review these changes, it is useful to emphasize the relevance of these developments to the subject of consensus in ethics committees. One reason why courts were skeptical of such extrajudicial mechanisms was their lack of grounding in statutory law; but another reason was a concern about due process, or ensuring that the rights of all parties to a fair hearing were preserved. Now, the vicissitudes of decision making by individuals (such as judges) and small groups (such as juries and ethics committees) are precisely what due process in the law is designed to guard against. Unlike with juries, there is no tradition of due process to guard against ethics committee recommendations that emerge from the flawed inner workings of some small groups.

The President's Commission report and "Baby Doe"

According to my analysis, the greatest impetus for ethics committees came from the political system rather than the legal system. In 1983 the President's Commission published *Deciding to Forgo Life-Sustaining Treatment*. One recommendation was that institutions should establish procedures to protect the self-determination and well-being of patients who lack decision-making capacity. Ethics committees were suggested as one way to promote effective decision making in ethically challenging cases. Among their possible functions the President's Commission listed diagnostic and prognostic review, staff education, policy formulation, review of physician or surrogate decisions, and decision making about specific cases.[32]

The Commission has been criticized for including the error made by the *Quinlan* Court and for the suggestion that committees themselves can make decisions about a patient's treatment. In the words of one commentator: "[M]edicine was not designed to be practiced by a Committee."[33] But the Commission's list referred to possible functions only, and in fact the report points out the error of the *Quinlan* Court in not understanding exactly what it was supposedly recommending. As for the role of committees in decision making, that complex matter is the subject of this book. It is naive, however, to think that small groups (whether they are called committees or teams or conferences) do not already play an important role in medical decision making, as the sociological literature attests, and surely the Commission was not recommending a role for ethics committees in technical *medical* decisions. Again, this was the error in *Quinlan*.

If there is a legitimate basis for criticizing the President's Commission's remarks on ethics committees in *Deciding to Forgo Life-Sustaining Treatment*, it lies in the ambiguous treatment of committees as advisory panels or as decision makers. The text strongly suggests that an advisory role is preferable when it quotes with emphasis the testimony of an experienced ethicist and member of a committee: "The one overriding theme of our meetings has been: '*we make no decision.*'"[34] But the report then goes on to hold open the door for a more decisive role. My impression is that the Commission intended to allow the possibility that ethics committees could actually make decisions for specific patients when the only other option is going to court. The most likely situation in which there would be a stark choice between a court and the ethics committee is that of a terminally ill and incapacitated patient lacking directives or a surrogate. Rather than have the doctor take complete responsibility for patients under such circumstances, it seems sensible to ask an intrainstitutional body to represent the patient's interests. In fact, as we shall see later, this is essentially the arrangement that has been proposed in New York State.

A further regulatory impetus for ethics committees occurred shortly after the President's Commission report. In response to a highly publicized case of non-treatment of a newborn with Down syndrome, the secretary of the Department of Health and Human Services published guidelines encouraging health care facilities to establish ethics committees. These guidelines replaced far more aggressive regulations that at one point included federal investigators and telephone hot lines to report "discrimination" against handicapped infants. The 1984 amendments to the Child Abuse Prevention and Treatment Act require all states receiving federal funds for their child abuse prevention programs to have a mechanism for ensuring that their intensive care nurseries are not engaging in discriminatory practices. Some participating states have elected to require "infant ethics committees" in level-3 nurseries as a way of meeting this requirement. Significantly, some of these neonatal committees are called "infant care review committees," a name preferred by the Reagan administration since it seemed to deemphasize the "quality of life" decisions that some associate with the fields of ethics and bioethics.[35]

It is noteworthy that the impetus for ethics committees in the years following the court cases came not only from government but also from the self-regulation of the health care industry, mainly under the rubric of "quality assurance." In 1985 an American Hospital Association Special Committee on Biomedical Ethics asserted that health care institutions must create policies and procedures to deal with ethical issues in the care of patients.[36] More recently the Joint Commission for the Accreditation of Healthcare Organizations (JCAHO) has begun to require "mechanism(s) for the consideration of ethical issues arising in the care of patients and to provide education to caregivers and patients on ethical issues in health care."[37] Ethics committees are clearly not mandated by the letter of this vague requirement, which could apparently be satisfied with one or two public lectures on medical ethics a year. Nevertheless, such committees have become the favored way for institutions to respond to these various new guidelines and requirements. In the future institutions may not have the luxury of choice concerning the creation of an ethics committee nor of its design and functions.

Statutory authority for ethics committees

In a liberal society characterized by value pluralism, ethics committees are an attractive way for hospitals to manage complex and controversial questions, especially in the absence of a clear judicial alternative. Under these circumstances, and along with developments in patients' rights, continuing technological advances, and persistent problems in financing health care, a turn toward mandating ethics committees not only is unsurprising but may even be overdetermined. State legislatures have responded in various ways, mainly using committees for decisions concerning incompetent patients. In Maryland disagreements among family members of the same class, such as adult children, concerning the termination of life-sustaining treatment must be referred to an institution's ethics committee. New Jersey's hospital licensing standards require a hospital to have either an ethics committee or a prognosis committee. In Arizona, if the authorized surrogate is not available, the attending physician may make treatment decisions after obtaining an ethics committee's recommendations.[38]

Probably the proposal that would most extensively empower ethics committees is that of New York State. A state oriented toward activism and regulation, it is also home to a disproportionate number of hospitals and produces a large number of the nation's doctors. New York would not only require committees of every hospital and nursing home but would establish specific responsibilities for them that would immunize other principals from legal liability. The requirement is part of a larger set of recommendations put forward by the Governor's Task Force on Life And the Law which concern decision making on behalf of incapacitated patients without advance directives or a durable power of attorney for health care. The recommendations were motivated by a lacuna in New York law between respect for the competent patient's wishes and deference to the decisions of a patient's previously appointed health care agent. The law has been such that incapacitated patients without an agent or clear and convincing prior statements concerning limiting treatment are subject to aggressive intervention regardless of the claims of family members about the patient's wishes.

Therefore, in 1992 the Task Force proposed that family members or close friends (according to a priority list) be recognized in the law as surrogates for patients. To provide some public assurance and accountability that surrogates are acting in good faith, all decisions to forgo life-sustaining treatment for non-dying patients would be subject to retrospective review by a facility-based "bioethics review committee." The structure and general procedures for the committee were also set forth in the bill, including multidisciplinary membership, a provision closely tied to usually unexamined philosophical assumptions about the importance of social diversity for morally valid consensus decisions. For patients who have no surrogate, the ethics committee itself makes decisions concerning the termination of life-sustaining treatment. Also noteworthy, and reminiscent of the IRB experience, is that the New York legislation specifies two ethical standards according to which surrogates and ethics committees are supposed to proceed: decisions are to be made either according to the likely wishes of the patient, so far as they can be known, or, failing that, in the best interests of the patient.[39]

With the New York proposal the history of ethics committees may yet reach its logical extreme in their entrenchment as another layer of legally required procedural decision making in the clinical, as against research, setting. The task force clearly hoped that its bioethics review committees would come to be accepted in their facility-based role on analogy with IRBs. Once created by the medical profession as a consultative mechanism composed entirely of physicians, committees that took a role in clinical ethics review have gradually acquired more regulatory authority and (owing to the widely perceived nonscientific element of moral decisions) have become less dominated by the medical profession.

Where, in all this, can one locate the importance of consensus? I have alluded to the political convenience of a committee process, but perhaps these committees would be just as legitimate socially if they always took a vote. In fact, I think, this is not the case. For the sake of argument, suppose that it turns out to be politically acceptable for IRBs to operate according to majority rule; after all, they could be (wrongly) perceived to be engaged in more "scientific" and "objective" issues than ethics committees, which are generally regarded as involved in factually "soft" and "fuzzy" questions. I contend that if it were not assumed that their deliberations are consensus-oriented, ethics committees would in point of fact be a far less acceptable social and political solution to the process of sorting out health care ethics than they have proven to be.

This contention returns me again to the summary view of ethics commissions in the previous chapter. In both cases the strength and weakness of consensus is precisely its tendency to obscure dissent. So much more important is it, therefore, for the field of bioethics to examine what goes on "inside" the ethics committee, and in particular to be aware of the dynamics of ethics committees as a kind of small group. We are also returned to the troubling question that arose with respect to ethics commissions. I have argued that the rise of ethics committees has been mostly due to their usefulness as instruments for the management of social controversy, and that their consensus orientation follows directly from this role. I have also contended that liberal political philosophy does not always provide straightforward validation of the moral authority of their consensus with respect to highly articulated issues. Under such circumstances the validation of moral consensus may turn on the extent to which the principles that are the objects of an overlapping consensus have been honored in the process. Thus the empirical background of consensus expressed in terms of actual social practices is all the more important. As in the case of ethics commissions, the political rationale for the authority of moral consensus seems to require the kind of supplementation that I will begin to provide in the next chapter.

Notes

1. President's Commission, *Deciding to Forgo Life-Sustaining Treatment*, p. 161.
2. "Hospital Ethics Committees Surveyed," *Hospitals* 58, 10 (1984): 52.
3. "Ethics Committees Double Since '83: Survey," *Hospitals* 59, 21 (1985): 64.
4. Brian S. Carter, "Medical Ethics Committees—A Survey of Army Hospitals," *Military Medicine* 153 (August 1988): 426–27.

5. Jonathan D. Moreno, "Who's to Choose? Surrogate Decision Making in New York State," *Hastings Center Report* 23, 1 (1993): 5–11.

6. Joint Commission on the Accreditation of Healthcare Organizations, "Patients' Rights," in *Accreditation Manual for Hospitals, 1992* (Chicago: JCAHO, 1992), pp. 103–105.

7. Diane E. Hoffmann, "Does Legislating Hospital Ethics Committees Make a Difference? A Study of Hospital Ethics Committees in Maryland, the District of Columbia, and Virginia," *Law, Medicine, and Health Care* 19, 1–2 (1991): 111.

8. See, for example, Stanley, *Technological Conscience*, p. 102.

9. Bernard Lo, "Behind Closed Doors: Promises and Pitfalls of an Ethics Committee," *New England Journal of Medicine* 317, 1 (1987): 46–49.

10. Jonathan D. Moreno, "Ethics Committees: Proceed with Caution," *Maryland Law Review* 50, 3 (1991): 895–903.

11. Ruth Macklin, "The Inner Workings of an Ethics Committee," *Hastings Center Report* 18, 1 (1998): 15–20.

12. *In re Quinlan* 355 A.2d 647 (N.J. 1976), *cert. denied*, 427 U.S. 1992 (1976).

13. Moreno, "Who's to Choose? Surrogate Decision Making in New York State," pp. 5–11.

14. Memo from Associate Chief for Program Development to Director, National Institutes of Health. "Progress Report on Survey of Moral and Ethical Aspects of Clinical Investigation." November 4, 1964, p. 6.

15. *Buck v. Bell*, 274 U.S. 200 (1927).

16. J. H. Landman, *Human Sterilization* (New York: Macmillan, 1932).

17. Robert Goldberg, Association for Voluntary Surgical Contraception, International. Personal communication, September 9, 1994. For a discussion of this issue see Richard K. Sherlock and Robert D. Sherlock, "Sterilizing the Retarded: Constitutional, Statutory and Policy Alternatives," *North Carolina Law Review* 60, 5 (1982): 943–83.

18. Landman, *Human Sterilization*, pp. 271–72.

19. Betty Sarvis and Hyman Rodman, *The Abortion Controversy* (New York: Columbia University Press, 1973).

20. Howard Hammond, "Therapeutic Abortion: Ten Years' Experience with Hospital Committee Control," *American Journal of Obstetrics and Gynecology* 89, 3 (1964): 352–53.

21. Sarvis and Rodman, *The Abortion Controversy*, p. 42.

22. Keith P. Russell, "Discussion of 'Therapeutic Abortion: Ten Years' Experience with Hospital Committee Control,'" *American Journal of Obstetrics and Gynecology* 89, 3 (1964): 352.

23. Shana Alexander, "They Decide Who Lives, Who Dies," *Life*, November 9, 1962. p. 102.

24. Department of Health and Human Services, "Rules and Regulations for Institutional Review Boards," *Federal Register* 45, 16 (1981): 8375.

25. Ibid.

26. Department of Health and Human Services, "Non-Local IRB Review," memorandum, January 1983, pp. 1–2.

27. Karen Teel, cited in *In re Quinlan*.

28. *In re Quinlan*.

29. *Superintendent of Belchertown State School v. Saikewicz*, 370 N.E. 2d 417 (Mass. 1977).

30. *In re Storar*, 420 N.E. 2d 64 (N.Y. 1981), *rev'd., In re Storar*, 443 N.Y.S. 2d 388 (App. Div. 1980), *aff'd., Eichner v. Dillon*, 426 N.Y.S. 2d 517 (App. Div. 1980).

31. *In re Colyer*, 660 P.2d 738 (Wash. 1983).

32. President's Commission, *Deciding to Forgo Life-Sustaining Treatment*.

33. Robert H. Sweeney, "Past, Present, and Future of Hospital Ethics Committees," *Delaware Medical Journal* 59, 3 (1987): 183.

34. President's Commission, *Deciding to Forgo Life-Sustaining Treatment*, p. 163.

35. Jonathan D. Moreno, "Ethical and Legal Issues in the Treatment of Impaired Newborns," *Clinics in Perinatology* 14, 2 (1987): 325–39.

36. *Values in Conflict: Resolving Ethical Dilemmas in Hospital Care* (Chicago: American Hospital Association, 1985).

37. Joint Commission, "Patients' Rights," p. 104.

38. Reported in Fletcher and Hoffmann, "Ethics Committees: Time to Experiment with Standards," p. 335.

39. Moreno, "Who's to Choose? Surrogate Decision Making in New York State."

7

Naturalizing Moral Consensus

Beyond the political rationale

In general, the lesson of the two preceding chapters is that it is reasonable to worry about the morality of the results of consensus processes that a liberal society may authorize, even if those processes appear to be in accord with the political rationale. The danger that consensus may obscure legitimate dissent and that consensus-oriented ethics panels may be politicized in a pejorative sense highlights worries about the morality of a particular consensus. Thus, we need to learn more about particular consensus processes to see if they sufficiently respect individual self-determination and other principles that are the objects of a society's settled overlapping consensus.

Even if these conditions are satisfied, there is a further question that the political rationale does not settle in and of itself: Is a particular moral consensus merely a matter of convention, or is it based on something that makes it more than a matter of collective human decision? After all, a moral consensus may meet political conditions such as respect for personal autonomy and still have its moral goodness challenged. The political rationale leaves other questions unanswered as well: How does consensus actually emerge from ethically problematic situations? What are the psychological and sociological conditions that make consensus possible? What does consensus look like in "real world" situations? These are among the questions I address in this chapter by developing a philosophy of moral consensus and by presenting three clinical sites for witnessing actual consensus processes.

My approach to these questions is indebted to a certain historic movement in philosophy called *naturalism*. Aristotle is the classical source of the naturalistic sensibility in philosophy, but the tradition has most recently been identified with American philosophers, especially John Dewey. Naturalism is essentially the view that values are not imposed from outside human experience but emerge from within it. According to this philosophy, moral consensus can be understood in natural terms, without an appeal to a transcendent moral order, and it is not accidental but explicable by appeal to empirical data. These data can be provided by the social sciences, literature, the arts, and indeed any field in which values are represented, for the act of representation is made possible by expression in symbols whose meanings are available to a community of understanding, meanings that reflect human experience. What might be called bioethical naturalism is a view of bioethics seen through the lens of naturalism. According to bioethical naturalism, the processes of bioethical consensus and the values embodied in it are part of human experience and are explicable in empirical terms.[1]

Toward a bioethical naturalism

Bioethical naturalism can provide an account of how a new moral consensus can emerge or, to use the language of the political rationale, how in a liberal and pluralistic society an overlapping consensus can stretch to manage novel cases and problems. This is possible because our ideas about the good life are not limited to a timeless set of moral truths that can subsist in a supernatural realm independent of human experience; instead they are part of the fabric of experience. As such our values are continuously brought to bear upon situations both old and new and are refined in light of those experiences. Although societal subgroups may subscribe to various comprehensive systems of belief, in pragmatic fact they adjust to more or less similar situations in ways that are not usually incompatible with one another, and even the relatively rare incompatibilities can also be empirically explained.

Bioethical naturalism as I conceive it is a philosophy *of* bioethics, a "metaphilosophy," and not a bioethical theory. In other words, it is an account of the generic nature of bioethics, not a competitor with ethical theories based on consequences or duties or bioethical methods based on principles, casuistry, virtue ethics, the ethics of care, or feminism. Whether bioethical naturalism is compelling or not, the liberal philosophy that provides a political rationale for the authority of consensus in a democratic society is independent of bioethical naturalism. At the same time, I believe that bioethical naturalism is in the same intellectual spirit as political liberalism. But naturalism pays special attention to the question of how moral consensus in fact emerges from problematic situations and how consensus processes can be better and worse, how ethical principles can be validly extended and how they can be distorted.

On one subject, however, naturalists part company with many political liberals, who often understand the principles about which there is moral consensus as merely conventional. To use the categories introduced in chapter 3, these liberals are intersubjectivists in their moral epistemology. For example, social contract theorists, for whom some original hypothetical contractors are projected as having reached an agreement that can be rationally reconstructed, tend to be conventionalists. Not all conventionalists are social contract theorists. Perhaps the most celebrated and consistent contemporary advocate of conventionalism in ethics is Richard Rorty, who has identified himself with other elements of the pragmatic tradition in philosophy. As a naturalist I concur with Rorty's rejection of transcendental moral absolutes (called objectivism in chapter 3) but not his evident lack of interest in the data of actual moral experience. As a naturalist I can live with Rorty's conclusion that, lacking a transcendent basis for morality, the best a civilized person can do is adopt an ironic posture. But I think Rorty underestimates the rich resources within human moral experience, and therefore overestimates the importance of an ironic attitude toward even the most treasured moral values.

Thus, I reject both absolutism and conventionalism as explanations of the nature of human morality.[2] As a naturalist I believe that there is a basis for moral consensus that is more than a matter of convention, that is integral to human experience. The data of moral psychology constitute part of my naturalistic view of moral consensus. These data suggest that there is a common moral sense that underlies human social arrangements. Furthermore, the idea of a common moral sense helps us to understand how a moral consensus can validly be extended in the light of new cases and problems.

Naturalists frequently appeal to empirical data as the basis for philosophical generalization; indeed, they often argue that philosophers have ignored the data of human experience, to their detriment. In *Experience and Nature* Dewey called on anthropological data for information about the general features of human existence, concluding from the universality of "sayings, proverbs and apothegms concerning luck" that instability and uncertainty are among the generic traits of human experience.[3] Although I am very sympathetic to this critique of philosophy in general, my aims in this book are far more limited than providing a generic account of human experience. Rather, my interest in naturalism is for its potential as a philosophical account of the possibility of moral consensus, an account that appeals to the data of human moral psychology.

Although naturalism resists obvious categorization according to the scheme of subjectivism, intersubjectivism, and objectivism introduced in chapter 3, there are certain difficulties for a naturalist in ethics. One is the so-called naturalistic fallacy, the illicit deduction of an "ought" or value statement from an "is" or fact statement. That is, merely because some people can be described as behaving in some way does not imply that they *ought* to behave in that way. But as the contemporary ethical naturalist Owen Flanagan notes concerning the alleged is-ought problem, no deduction of ethical truths from descriptions of conduct need be attempted. "[T]he smart naturalist makes no claims to establish demonstratively moral norms—he or she points to certain practices as wise or reasonable based on inductive and abductive reasoning."[4] In any case, the idea of the moral sense to which I appeal does not lend support to particular moral judgments, though it is suggestive of certain tendencies in conduct.

A second difficulty for a naturalist is the prospect that some empirical generalizations about human moral behavior will turn out to be highly contextual with regard to time and place. Those who appeal to a moral sense must beware of ethno- and era-centrism. As an ethical naturalist I am prepared to accept the fact that the ends of ethics are both geographically and temporally local, that ethical inquiry differs from scientific inquiry in this respect.[5]

Most of the rest of this chapter is concerned with the empirical and philosophical elements of this naturalistic view of moral consensus. First, however, I want to return to the history of the idea of moral consensus, this time emphasizing the naturalism that has repeatedly turned up in its history. Of course, historical analysis does not in itself settle the question of how moral consensus should be understood, but it does demonstrate that naturalism is no stranger to the idea of consensus.

The naturalistic roots of consensus

The history of the idea of consensus reveals that the understanding of consensus has repeatedly returned to a naturalistic philosophy as against a notion of consensus as a matter of mere convention. As we shall see, this has been particularly true when an organismic conception of society has prevailed. Furthermore, at some point *moral* consensus was separated from the more general concept, and it remained for American pragmatists to reassert the unity of the consensus idea.

Percy Herbert Partridge has characterized the ideas of consent and consensus as "persistent and elusive" throughout intellectual history,

persistent, because there have been thinkers in all times who have held that there must be an element of agreement or consensus in the constitution of human society; and elusive, because these thinkers have always found it difficult to specify what the nature of that consensus may be.[6]

There is, however, an aspect of the consensus idea that surfaces repeatedly in its history. Ancient writers, including especially Plato, Aristotle, and Cicero, resisted merely conventional explanations of the basis for social organization. The ancients tended instead to emphasize naturalistic or biological grounds for the entrance of individuals into civil society, roughly on the model of the family. Needs for food, shelter, and a primitive division of labor supposedly prompted the first moment of social organization. This view furthermore gives a virtually organic cast to civil society as a system whose parts are functionally related. Classical authorities did not regard *consent* as a sufficiently powerful device to account for the origin of civil life. They did, however, regard *consensus* as an important part of the ongoing character of social relations, which they conceived in organic terms.

In part because of a theology that was sympathetic to the idea of social agreement, and in part because of the ancient recognition of popular agreement as essential for social unity, early medieval kings were constrained by a primitive notion of contract whereby regal authority was assured so long as the requirements of the lords and other powerful men were respected. In the sixteenth and seventeenth centuries, when rulers insisted on their "divine right," the underdeveloped notion of consent of the governed was sharpened into its recognizably modern form which sees each individual as a rights holder.

Consensus, as distinguished from consent, appears to have emerged in the modern period as part of an account of the ongoing cohesiveness of civil society, following the theoretical acceptance of a social contract. Hooker alluded to the "silent allowances" that manifest themselves in so many individuals' continuing loyalty to all sorts of customs, as against the "express consent" that produces "positive laws." In Locke the concept of "tacit consent" includes that of continuous though unstated obedience to government. It is important to note that these writings which prefigured more recent talk of consensus reintroduce the ancient naturalistic or organismic picture of civil society. Thus J. S. Mill followed Comte in defining consensus as the mutual influence of every part of society on every other part.

It was, however, the Scottish rather than the English philosophers who preserved a dynamic concept of the human actor. In spite of Locke's appreciation of the social dimension, his philosophy did not provide a rich explanation of the human capacity for moral and aesthetic experience. The forward-looking and influential earl of Shaftesbury, writing in the early eighteenth century, looked to empirical psychology for answers to Hobbes's egoistic characterization of human beings. Shaftesbury held that social affections are just as natural in humankind as self-regarding affections; thus, disinterested benevolence is essential for human happiness. Significant for my purposes is the idea of social affections, for these are implicitly universal, or very nearly so, and they express themselves in social relations. In chapter 4 I mentioned Shaftesbury's chief successor, Francis Hutcheson, founder of the moral sense school, which continued to emphasize the role of psychology in ethics. I also mentioned the Scottish realists, who were so important to the philosophy that gave shape to the thinking of the American founders. Their most tangible legacy is the idea of the self-evidence of moral truths, supposedly derived from an immediate intellectual insight. Unlike traditional moral sense theory, however, the modern variety relies on evidence from empirical studies of human behavior rather than intellectual insight or intuition.

The psychology of moral consensus

According to liberal political philosophy the validity of a moral consensus depends partly on the extent to which certain values have been respected in the deliberative process. These values include respect for the individual and an openness to alternative points of view. Since, as a bioethical naturalist, I reject the view that any resulting consensus either is merely a matter of convention or has some transcendental standing, I need to explain how it is possible for disparate individuals to achieve moral agreement. How is moral consensus between persons even possible in the first place if it is not either arbitrary or dictated by some eternal Truth? An answer is especially important for a field such as bioethics, which trades in novel ethical problems. If we had a psychological theory that could account for consensus formation among discrete individuals, we would be well on the way to answering this question.

The psychology of moral consensus was prefigured in my mention of the moral sense school of eighteenth-century Scottish philosophy, a tradition that includes famous figures such as Adam Smith and David Hume as well as less famous ones such as Francis Hutcheson. James Q. Wilson has recently attempted to extend this tradition, which holds that there is a moral sense that is virtually universal among human beings, by comparing its key contention with the findings of modern social science. If the moral sense claim can be thus sustained, it would represent an empirical basis for morality, which could inform a naturalistic ethics. That is, instead of offering a justification of a set of moral rules, the theory of moral sense provides a description of a set of moral perceptions—perceptions that are inferred from the study of human behavior. Of particular interest for my project, since virtually all human beings are alleged to possess this moral sense, it could provide the basis for an empirical explanation of the possibility of moral consensus.[7]

Wilson's argument proceeds on the basis of a considerable body of psychological evidence, of which a couple of examples will suffice. He points to a remarkable uniformity in human reactions to another individual in distress, in that if people are part of a crowd, they tend not to intervene, whereas a sole witness will tend to come to the sufferer's aid. Explanations for the failure to intervene are many, including a lessened feeling of individual responsibility, but the conditions associated with intervention indicate altruism, for the helpful lone bystander acts in spite of the absence of approving witnesses. Wilson relates this uniform result to the sociable virtue that Adam Smith called sympathy.[8]

In another example, studies of behavior among children indicate an easy familiarity with the virtue of fairness by age four. That is, even if children do not always exhibit fairness themselves, they are able to call upon the idea of sharing and protest when they perceive an inequity. Especially interesting is that in adults the sense of fairness is perceptible in contrast to rational self-interest. Wilson describes studies that involve a two-player game called Ultimatum, in which the first player is given some money, say ten dollars, which may be shared in any way he or she desires, knowing both that there will not be another round and that the game will never be played again. Rationality suggests that the first player should give away only one cent and keep the rest, but what usually happens is that the first player proposes either an equal division or around a 70–30 split, even though there is nothing for the first player to gain in so doing. Furthermore, even though the second player has nothing to lose by taking whatever is offered, lopsided offers tend to be rejected.[9]

Many elements of Wilson's argument are relevant to naturalism in ethics, such as the role of evolution in the selection of traits such as sympathy and fairness.[10] The importance of these sorts of results for a theory of moral consensus lies in their ability to account for the fact that individuals tend to agree about right and wrong. There are, of course, various possible objections to the conclusions Wilson draws. For instance, one can attempt to cite counterexamples from anthropological fieldwork to the effect that these and other traits are not universally manifested. Wilson contends that these results are universal enough to stand up to anthropological evidence. The ethical naturalist is, as I have said, prepared to accept that ethics will not in all specifics be universal. Or one could hold up as a counterexample to the idea of a shared moral sense the widespread existence of criminality. Wilson's reply is that, demographically, the proportion of serious offenders has not varied much from one time or society to another, and that even most career criminals say they would be "very angry" if one of their children were to commit a crime.[11] In any case, my job as a philosopher is not to defend the reliability of this information. But as a naturalist, to the extent that it provides an empirical basis for philosophical theorizing, I cannot ignore it.

The evidence also suggests that, when children learn about morality, they tend to learn about the same thing. In the words of the pragmatic philosopher Paul Churchland:

Young children learn to recognize a distribution of scarce resources such as cookies or candies as a *fair* or *unfair distribution*. They learn to voice complaint in the latter case, and to withhold complaint in the former. They learn to recognize that a found object may be *someone's property*, and that access is limited as a result. They learn to discriminate *unprovoked cruelty*, and to demand or expect punishment for the transgressor and comfort for the victim. They learn to recognize a *breach of promise*, and to howl in protest. They learn to recognize these and a hundred other prototypical social/moral situations, and the ways in which the embedding society generally reacts to those situations and expects them to react. . . . What the child is learning in this process is the *structure of social space* and *how best to navigate one's way through it*. What the child is learning is practical wisdom: the wise administration of her practical affairs in a complex social environment. This is as genuine a case of learning about objective reality as one finds anywhere.[12]

All this leads one to conclude that children both learn and are prepared to learn certain facts about morality; through this interaction the moral sense becomes visible: and the commonality of this experience of moral development can be identified as a shared moral sense.

A shared moral sense, however, is not tantamount to a shared moral justification. As the logicians would say, sense is not isomorphic to judgment or belief; there is "logical slack" between the moral sense and particular expressions of moral approval and disapproval. For example, in ethical theory utilitarians and deontologists vehemently disagree, but their disagreements are often about how best to justify propositions about which they share a moral sense, such as that doctors should respect the wishes of the patient with capacity. When they are spinning out their different justifications for these sorts of judgments (in search of a deep consensus), utilitarianism and deontology sound pretty good. But when they enter territory in which the moral sense is less reliable, such as the morality of abortion, ethical theories that seemed muscular when the conclusion to be justified was uncontroversial appear impotent when it is a matter of heated debate.

Thus, it would be a mistake to conclude that the principles that are the objects of an overlapping consensus in a pluralistic society, taken together, constitute the moral sense. It would also be erroneous to think that there are different items in the moral sense that correspond to individual principles endorsed by the overlapping consensus. The moral sense does not work that way. But it does tend toward certain principles and away from others, and these tendencies are represented in the principles that are accepted by a liberal society which respects the individual as possessed of a moral sensibility and, therefore, entitled to be respected as a being with moral value.

A naturalistic philosophy of moral consensus

I have argued that a satisfactory account of moral consensus in a pluralistic society can be achieved only if philosophical liberalism is supplemented. Once it is agreed that the study of actual consensus processes is needed to understand how moral consensus is in fact possible, or to understand how, in a pluralistic society, a bioethical moral consensus can be validly extended to novel cases and problems, we are well on the way to what I call the naturalization of moral consensus. In the previous sections I approached the naturalization of moral consensus as a matter of the history of ideas and of psychological explanation; in subsequent discussions I approach it in terms of small group processes. In this section I treat it at a generic, philosophical level.

As a naturalist I hold that moral values emerge from actual human experience and are not superimposed on it by some transcendental reality (Plato's Forms are the classic example). Thus I believe we cannot learn about moral consensus or improve arrangements aimed at extending it without at least looking toward actual consensus processes. From the standpoint of ethical naturalism the hypothesis of the moral sense, and the evidence that Wilson and others have gathered for it, accounts for the possibility of a shared moral sense.

Earlier I suggested that a consensus not only marks a specific conclusion but, more important, has to do with a process of decision making. Thus, the term does not identify a discrete and wholly unambiguous idea or refer to a precise end point of deliberation but rather alludes to a deliberative process. Nor, in fact, does this process have a distinct beginning, for the countless assumptions that underlie and qualify the process are themselves a latent consensus. From the perspective of political philosophy they are the principles in the overlapping consensus; from the naturalistic perspective they are dispositions whose origins are lost in the antiquity of social relations and human evolution. We should be careful not to allow ourselves to be taken in by certain common ways of talking about consensus, that we "seek" it or that it is something that is "reached." According to a naturalistic account of consensus, it is not merely the product of deliberation (an abstract goal) but rather an integral part of the deliberative process itself. In a naturalistic philosophy of consensus the first commandment is, "Thou shalt not hypostatize consensus!"

Besides alerting us to the confusions inherent in treating consensus as a mere product of moral deliberation, a naturalistic philosophy of consensus also deepens understanding of the generic features of consensus. In the first place, consensus processes are inextricably associated with inquiry, and inquiry takes place when a problematic situation is encountered. A reliable indication that a problematic situation has been encountered is a feeling of doubt that prior assumptions are adequate in the management of a current "state of affairs."[13] In general, a state of affairs is a dynamic situation, with disparate elements or energies in play. Some of these energies are relatively stable (a state), while others are in relative flux (affairs). Fortunately, no state of affairs is ever either wholly stable (for then change would be impossible) or wholly in flux (for then management would be impossible). The issue of a state of affairs is the theme that emerges from the interplay of stable and changing elements. By a solution to the issue of a state of affairs is meant a conclusion that brings the elements into a satisfactory relationship with one another.

Although this philosophical account of states of affairs seems at first rather vague and puzzling, it does square with our subjective experience. A musical analogue of this philosophy of states of affairs is jazz, which helps explain why so many have taken jazz to be the musical genre that most closely reflects the experience of subjectivity. Jazz has stable and changing elements, and at a certain point in this unfolding structure a theme emerges. How the theme is finally resolved with respect to the elements of the structure from which it emerged determines whether the piece succeeds or not, and that is determined by the success of the "solution" in making sense of the musical images that appeared in uncertain relation to one another earlier in the work.

Readers who do not consider themselves jazz buffs might instead think about a favorite novel, film, or play. Relatively stable elements in the tale, such as certain features of the characters' personalities, are established, and these coexist with changing elements such as the series of situations the characters face. The aesthetic success of the work is partly determined by the way the themes appear to emerge integrally from the interplay of character and situation, and how well the climax "makes sense" in terms of what has gone before. Ultimately the successful work of literature is one that has an "end" rather than one that only finishes; the former sort of work involves a satisfying conclusion that gives meaning to the whole and seems well suited to it, whereas the latter fails to have a meaning and often leaves the audience frustrated and disappointed.

Let me see if I can cash in this naturalistic account of states of affairs by applying it to an analysis of what is meant by a "case." As that term is used in medicine, law, or ethics, it is not very well defined, but our implicit understanding of it does bear marked similarities to the idea of a state of affairs in a naturalistic philosophy. That is, there are familiar and stable elements of a case (the relevant biomedical theory, the available interventions, the goals of therapy), and there are unstable elements (the possibility of alternative explanations, the prospect for efficacious treatment, the patient's ability to cope with therapy). As the case unfolds, certain primary and secondary issues or themes emerge (the likely benefit to the patient of one or another management strategy, the risks of innovative treatment). Finally, the approach taken in the attempt to manage these disparate elements may give them collective meaning (which implies nothing about the outcome for the patient, which may be good or bad).

We can return now to the idea of the problematic situation that is encountered as part of a state of affairs. In her effort to resolve the problem, the inquirer must call on various resources, both "internal" (her ingenuity, patience, and other such personal qualities) and "external" (the relatively stable features of the state of affairs, including available theories and technologies). A useful idea at this stage is that of evaluation, literally, "drawing the value from." In assessing her situation the inquirer draws from it both moral and nonmoral values that are inherent in the state of affairs. These values will give shape and direction to her formulation and implementation of a proposed solution. If, for example, the problematic situation involves whether or not to recommend chemotherapy to a cancer patient, an evaluation will include the identification of the most appropriate medications and dosage (a nonmoral value) and the likelihood of benefit for this patient (a moral value).[14]

Now add to this naturalistic account of a case the idea of a community of inquirers (of which our democratic deliberators are an example). All human endeavors have an ineluctably social dimension, and the operation of science and other forms of systematic inquiry, such as ethics, depend on cooperation. Furthermore, although I have used the clinical case as an example, any problematic situation has the same generic properties. Evaluation of a problematic situation by an ethics panel entails the drawing out of values that may not be equally apparent from all points of view, which is precisely why various viewpoints are desirable. Because of differences in disciplinary training, cultural background, age, sex, or other factors, the attention of different group members is directed in different ways. The constructive exploitation of these differences through collaborative inquiry is the exercise of what has been called social intelligence.[15]

The exercise of social intelligence, of cooperation in inquiry by disparate individuals, each with her own goals and attitudes, is perhaps easier said than done. Still, cynicism should be tempered by the record, for while history records countless examples of abject stupidity and cruelty, it also indicates occasions of intelligent action and human solidarity. It is awfully hard to articulate just what it is that enables individuals together to achieve breakthroughs that they could not have achieved separately. Part of the answer is the economy of group activity, but another part is surely the richness, and attendant complexity, that various participants can bring to the table. In social affairs, perhaps unlike theoretical science, there is the further need to formulate a common acceptable framework for the resolution of moral controversy, one that will be much harder to forge in isolation.

Uncertainty in the face of a problematic situation is essential both for a condition of authentic cooperative inquiry and for the possibility that a consensus will emerge. Uncertainty is first and foremost that which distinguishes a matter of genuine concern from a mere intellectual exercise. But what sets consensus apart from compromise is, as I pointed out in chapter 2, precisely that in consensus the participants enter the scene in doubt about how to resolve the problem, whereas in compromise the participants have no doubts, except perhaps about how best to ensure that their position largely prevails. Uncertainty is therefore a precondition for sincere inquiry and helps establish the conditions for a level of openness to others; its absence guarantees a degree of posturing and "politics" in the pejorative sense.

The idea of consensus as "emergent" deserves further comment. Emergence is an important notion for naturalists because it suggests that no situations are wholly new; they share more or less enduring characteristics with those that came before and those that come later. In the natural world change has both dynamic and static elements. Situations are therefore always relatively novel, some more than others. Among the enduring features of a novel situation are ordinarily some values that might be brought to bear, such as the principles that are the objects of an overlapping consensus. Thus, while a particular new situation might well constitute an "emergency" in that it creates conditions that must be addressed at the earliest practical time, it will still contain some features that are somewhat familiar. Were this not the case, then it could not successfully be dealt with at all.

A crucial element in the passage from uncertainty to the satisfactory management of a problematic situation is that the proposed solution or hypothesis must be seen as a reasonable one in light of the available evidence. Naturalists and other pragmatists, especially including those known as "experimentalists," call this *warranted assertability*, a phrase that Dewey proposed to explicate the transcendent-sounding word *truth*. For example, the hypothesis that there is a moral sense, if accepted by the relevant community of inquirers, should be regarded as warrantedly assertable just insofar as it plays a satisfactory role in the management of information about human behavior. Similarly, that there is an obligation to respect the wishes of competent patients should be viewed as a warranted assertion about medical ethics rather than a transcendental moral truth.[16]

In summary, according to a naturalistic account of the role of consensus in ethics, the point of ethical deliberation is not to "reach consensus" per se but to bring a controversy to some desirable (if always tentative) conclusion. Along the way there must be agreement about the soundness of the method being used. Thus, consensus is not an abstract end but is itself an activity, a process. In turn, consensus conditions a process of cooperative and intelligent reconstruction of a troubling situation into one in which whatever latent values there are can be recognized and, by taking some action, perhaps more fully enjoyed. The proposed way in which this is to be done is a hypothesis, subject to change in the light of experience with its applications. The hypothesis must continually meet the challenge of warranted assertability, and it does this to the extent that evidence on its behalf continues to be persuasive to the community of inquirers.

Witnessing consensus processes in the clinic

This abstract account of consensus processes can be brought down to earth by "witnessing" situations in which moral consensus plays a critical role. For a naturalist, examples like the ones I am about to present are important because they show how moral consensus processes are integral elements of human affairs, even those that are closely bound up with scientific matters.

In sociological terms consensus can be understood in part as a form of social control. There is nothing insidious about this idea. Consensus helps to organize and coordinate the energies of individual human beings, especially those who must work closely together in order to meet social goals. As I observed earlier, the study of societal consensus has long been an important part of the sociologist's trade. More recently sociology has placed a greater emphasis on the inherently political nature of human institutions. Sociologists have tended to emphasize the ways in which interpersonal systems are influenced by power relations rather than by more general phenomena of acquiescence and assent.

Although it is admittedly not the rational process that was envisioned by the Enlightenment philosophers who were inspired by classical thought, consensus as social control does important work. From the point of view of political sociology, even the oldest known consensus document in the history of medicine, the Hippocratic oath in its various versions, can be viewed as a mechanism for social control. Indeed, in principle all oaths are intended to bind individuals organically as members (a revealingly anatomical term) of the cult or fraternity, and Hippocratists were bound by the adoption of certain values and modes of conduct. Some aspects of the Hippocratic consensus have had remarkable staying power and remain part of the moral consensus of physician conduct, such as the ban on sexual contact with patients. Others have fallen away as the new medical ethics has displaced the old, such as the wholesale legitimacy of therapeutic privilege.

To be sure, one important functional difference between the Hippocratic oath in its original context and as a vestigial part of modern medical school commencement exercises is the fact that in the ancient world it served to distinguish the Hippocratists from other ancient physicians. The consensus of an "in-group" is obviously much sharper and more immediately bound up with its survival than is the consensus of a group that has no serious competition in the medical marketplace, as is the case for contemporary scientific medicine. However, in either case the specifics of the consensus remain terribly important in the control of members' behavior and in the way that these initiated individuals view their realm of professional activity.

Again, to nonsociologists the notion of "social control" can be somewhat jarring. But the foundation of this idea is not dictatorship or conspiracy; rather, it is that of social stability and cohesion. A consensus can be an organizing principle for a group, a source of order and structured, purposeful activity. Thus, Partridge points out that much social behavior that conforms with custom or tradition can be counted as consensus. An exception would be a class of slaves who unthinkingly and unquestioningly perform customary roles. But, Partridge continues, "there are other cases . . . where people have come to feel that their traditions and customs have an inherent claim on their respect and obedience." The institutions of medicine provide vivid examples of this. Consensus can thus be seen as involving "an intellectual or emotional relation to the object which may be justly characterized as *agreement* with it."[17]

The Hippocratic oath, or its functional equivalents in other cultures, helps define the social territory of the medical profession generally. Specialties within medicine have their own characteristic forms of self-regulation, many of which are far less formal but are nevertheless socially powerful. In the next three sections I briefly describe several examples of consensus processes as social control mechanisms in modern clinical medicine. All are derived from recent sociological literature and give eloquent testimony to the ways in which consensus is integral to the clinical context. To be sure, the examples I have chosen—the surgical morbidity and mortality conference,[18] the medical intensive care unit,[19] and the genetic counseling clinical conference[20]—are rather intensified versions of the more general insight about the role of consensus as a source of group stability even in the face of situations that threaten to disturb the group's cohesion. My debt to the sociological researchers Charles Bosk and Robert Zussman will be evident as I proceed.

One specific lesson of these examples turns out to be the motivation for consensus processes in modern medicine, as compared to its celebrated Hippocratic traditions. For whereas the Hippocratists were probably most concerned with managing group identity, modern applied medical scientists are most concerned with managing group uncertainty. This concern is probably more pronounced in those highly specialized fields that have a large stake in their scientific reputation. But even for modern medicine as a whole, this seems to be an important difference in the role of consensus processes in ancient Hippocratic medicine and in modern scientific medicine. The latter is characterized by dramatic interventions made reasonable by greater understanding of human physiology and biochemistry, and made technically possible by drugs and devices. By contrast, the most dramatic intervention available to the ancients, surgery, was explicitly proscribed in the Hippocratic consensus. Whether this and other checks on the practice of ancient physicians were actually effective is a separate question, but, as we shall see, there is little doubt that the uncertainties associated with the outcomes of modern medical interventions have resulted in powerful mechanisms of social control.

In addition to teaching us about consensus processes as elements of health care decision making, these case studies help us identify some important aspects of a more general understanding of actual consensus processes. And, beyond the social control aspects of consensus, it is important to note the way uncertainty creates a problematic situation that requires some form of resolution, as well as the role that values play in organizing group activity. These are two basic features of a naturalized view of emerging moral consensus.

Case Study 1: The Surgical Morbidity and Mortality Conference

A hallmark of medical sociology has long been the observation that uncertainty is an important issue for medical students, long before they undertake graduate medical education or medical practice. This "training for uncertainty" involves several distinct stages, including especially the student's willingness (by the end of undergraduate medical school) to accept the inherent uncertainty of this applied science and to proceed in spite of it. But this resolve is insufficient in specific cases without the support of peers who have also accepted the ironic attitude toward medical uncertainty. Thus, consensus is deeply rooted in the socialization of young physicians.

In his classic study of a surgical residency program, *Forgive and Remember*, Charles Bosk describes the ways in which the authority of the attending surgeon is legitimized. Focusing on the morbidity and mortality conference, Bosk offers a particularly intriguing pair of examples that show how the "working consensus of the group"[21] manifests itself—in one case by its glaring absence, in the other by its reinforcement at a time of crisis. The first example is one of failure of a treatment that was chosen from among other alternatives with equal prospects for success, and the second is one of failure of a statistically preferred alternative.

In the first example procedures A, B, and C all hold equally low prospects for success, and the burden is therefore on the attending surgeon to justify his or her choice of the alternative that is chosen regardless of a scientific basis for that or any other choice. When the procedure fails, it is in the morbidity and mortality conference that the attending, who is normally exempt from such humiliation rituals, must answer for the mistake. The conference is then transformed into a "seminar in abstract problem solving," as Bosk describes it. The attending "puts on the hair shirt" that is, takes total responsibility for the way the decision making was carried out, explains how the miscalculation occurred and how it will be corrected in the future. Bosk argues that an important feature of this ritual is to exemplify for the residents the way a senior surgeon shoulders the burdens of individual judgment.[22]

The surgical morbidity and mortality conference provides an extraordinary occasion in which to mark a lack of scientific and clinical consensus in such a case. It is in stark contrast to the ordinary course of clinical events, in which there are no such gross deviations from common agreement, and there is certainly no need for the eminences to don the hair shirt. By contrast, in the morbidity and mortality conference the customary working atmosphere of consensus is a Sartrean "present absence," as the attending places herself on the altar of self-criticism while subordinates look on in respectful silence.

In the second example of failure Bosk offers the statistically preferred alternative was selected, but grave consequences ensued anyway. This sort of failure is attributed not to the medical decision-making process itself but to the way in which the decision was implemented. Privately the attendings blame their subordinates, the house staff, but in the public setting of the morbidity and mortality conference they blame themselves for their negligence in failing to foresee a problem in execution, such as "inadequate" instruction of residents in certain technical procedures. As in the first example, the attendings model for their juniors the sort of individual responsibility that comes with the social privileges accorded surgeons. This exercise in humility also somewhat mitigates the daily harassment that these distinguished instructors level at the house officers as part of surgical education.

There are several dimensions of consensus at work in this second example from Bosk. First, there had been a consensus about the indicated surgical approach, one that is made obvious by the failure in this case. Second, there is an implicit consensus in this group that even prestigious surgeons should admit error in the presence of their subordinates, though in highly controlled conditions. Third, and perhaps most intriguing, part of the very process of the attending's self-criticism is supportive statements by other senior members of the group. As Bosk reports:

> The humbling effects [of the conference] are ordinarily softened, either by other attendings who indicate that they would have handled the case in the same way or who cite similar examples from their own clinical history or by pathologists who indicate that the patient was ravaged by disease and beyond repair.[23]

Thus, a philosophical working consensus of the group about the limits of surgical intervention is reinforced even as the ritual of self-criticism is played out.

Case Study 2: The Intensive Care Unit

The setting of the intensive care unit (ICU) has been described by Robert Zussman in *Intensive Care*. Here, too, there is a consensus about the nature of responsibility which must be passed on to physicians in training. But the demands of the ICU create a somewhat different sort of consensus from that of the surgical department. Whereas in surgery the emphasis is on hierarchy, ICU work leads to a great deal of mutual dependence, particularly among the residents. Thus, while the ICU attendings emphasize abstract obligations to patients, functionally for the house staff the focus is on responsibility to one another. In effect this amounts to the same thing, Zussman argues, but the immediate reaction to individual failure in the ICU is put in terms of shirking responsibility. Other residents and interns will punish this sort of behavior by not making the greater effort at assistance they might provide another peer. "Indeed," Zussman writes, "for the occasional intern or, even more rarely, resident who does not meet his or her responsibilities, the ICU rotation becomes a special and lonely misery."[24]

The uncertainty associated with treating patients who are gravely ill is, of course, an especially important factor in the ICU. Zussman notes that the normative consensus of medical ethics proscribes withdrawing or withholding treatment (aside from those who have made such a request), except from patients who are clearly terminal. Since prognostic certainty is hard to achieve in medicine generally, and because the stakes of being wrong are so high in intensive care, physicians tend to treat aggressively until the course of a patient's disease is understood. By this time we often discover, with the aid of a "retrospectorscope," that a patient has been subjected to considerable overtreatment. Again, since medicine is not a theoretical but an applied science, inductive uncertainty is pervasive.

To the essential nature of prognostic uncertainty are added several social factors that exacerbate the situation, according to Zussman. Among these is the responsibility of the individual physicians. As was the case for their counterparts in surgery, this hallowed tradition has clear implications for the consensus processes of intensive care medicine. So important is consensus among the intensivists that a single dissent is enough to create doubt. Indeed, Zussman's study of the ICU suggests that even a resident may successfully carry an argument to continue treatment while others object. This deviation from hierarchic authority is possible because of the fundamental commitment to preserve life unless the cause is hopeless, and "hopelessness" is determined, as a social matter, by the agreement of all members of the team that nothing more can be done. This combination of an emphasis on collective decision making in the ICU with that on individual physician responsibility renders decisions to limit treatment, as compared with decisions to continue treatment, terribly elusive.

Case Study 3 : **The Genetics Counseling Clinic**

Finally, in *All God's Mistakes* Bosk reports on his ethnographic work in a genetic counseling clinic. Much of his commentary has to do with a source of tension in the work of the counselors. Although the philosophy of genetic counseling emphasizes a nondirective approach and autonomy of the prospective parents, there was often consensus among the group of counselors Bosk studied about which conditions warranted abortion. When the counselors perceived themselves as unable to get through to a counselee how grave the situation was, they were frustrated that the ethos of the field did not permit them to go farther and directively counsel termination of pregnancy. In spite of these worries about seemingly unreasonable behavior by their patients, it is striking how religiously the counselors abided by their nondirective code.

Still more interesting were those occasions when the group's consensus broke down. In one such case one of the counselors had been working with a couple whose infant, stricken with multiple anomalies, had recently died. The counselor reassured the couple that their baby's condition was an accidental defect and not the result of a chromosomal anomaly. The embryologist had arrived at this conclusion, the counselor explained, because the defect occurred at a particular moment of the pregnancy rather than expressing itself throughout the entire pregnancy. The counselor thus strongly assured the couple that there was nothing they could have done to anticipate the problem, and no reason to think that it would happen in a subsequent pregnancy. During this discourse and at the end of the session the couple reacted with relief and gratitude.[25]

In the counselors' clinic conference the following day the counselor presented this couple's case. One of the other members asked if there was in fact evidence that because an event occurs at one point in embryo genesis, this shows it is not a result of genetic disease. The couple's counselor replied that there was no such evidence and confessed his discomfort that unconfirmed theories were being used as clinical guidelines in their counseling. Until the question was raised, Bosk observes, "it was not apparent that any uncertainty existed at all," reflecting a state of "pluralistic ignorance" in the group, as each member kept his or her own doubts private. Yet the question, when finally asked, created apprehension in the group: "The acknowledgment of uncertainty dissolved the group consensus and created great distrust of the clear directive 'not to worry' given to the patients."[26]

Moral consensus and natural habitats

I have offered these scenarios as examples of "natural habitats" in which informal consensus processes operate. Each is an illustration of the way problematic situations occur in the states of affairs characteristic of modern clinical medicine, and each issues a profound challenge to a socially intelligent response. Although the consensus processes implicit in these problematic situations are unsystematic (and the results not wholly admirable), an observer can nevertheless detect regular features and a sort of deliberateness.

The surgical unit, the intensive care unit, and the genetic counselors' clinic conference are perhaps not typical of the practice of medicine generally, where the stakes are normally not as high and colleagues do not work together so closely. Indeed, in some respects they probably have more in common with hospital ethics committees than with solo medical practice. Ethics committees, like departments of surgery, intensive care units, and counseling staffs, often deliberate as small groups on matters that involve considerable uncertainty and are associated with the most far-reaching consequences for those concerned. Given the importance of consensus elsewhere in the hospital, it is not surprising that these committees would adopt a posture about their own decision making that is familiar in the culture of health care.

Some useful generalizations about clinical consensus processes can be inferred from these case studies. I list only a few that are directly relevant to my concerns in this book. First, hierarchical structures, which are otherwise so important, can be rendered at least temporarily irrelevant for the sake of a more basic principle about which there is agreement. In the surgical conference and in the ICU the principle is the desirability of the best possible outcome for the patient. Second, those who fail to appreciate their mutual responsibilities are subject to harsh informal discipline by their peers. Here again a notion of equality is at work. Third, the emphasis on the autonomy of patients is greatest when there is uncertainty about the meaning of a "desirable outcome," as in the genetics counseling situation. Finally, as is especially common in genetics counseling but could also apply in surgery and the ICU, uncertainty about what counts as a desirable outcome is so powerful in the clinical setting that it can jeopardize the underlying consensus of the group about many other matters. There is an important lesson here about the significance of the principle of beneficence in the structure of beliefs that can support a clinical team's consensus.

At a still higher level of generality are the ways in which principles that are the object of an overlapping consensus in a liberal and diverse society, and liberal values, manifest themselves. In the morbidity and mortality conference equality is more important than hierarchy because the stakes are so high for future patients, though the equality can be so brutal that it is ritually modified by personal expressions of support. In the ICU status gives way to openness to alternative points of view, though admittedly a single dissent may feed an aggressive treatment philosophy that is open to question. Genetics counselors may feel so bereft of substantive principles to guide them in ethically novel territory that they fall back on the well-accepted but highly abstract procedural principle of personal autonomy. It comes as no surprise that, when a group defaults to principles about which there is a consensus, the results are not always unalloyed goods; the burden rests on those who would propose superior alternatives.

In these kinds of settings the importance of moral consensus is apparent in the way it organizes the activities and energies of diverse and highly skilled men and women, and also in the efforts that are made to repair the consensus once a problematic situation has been encountered. These examples help demonstrate the argument of this chapter: that moral consensus is a natural feature of human affairs, that it manifests itself in and emerges from social practices, and that human experience contains both the conditions that undermine the quality of a moral consensus and the resources that enable us to improve it.

Notes

1. For a classic collection of essays on philosophical naturalism, see Yervant H. Krikorian, ed., *Naturalism and the Human Spirit* (New York: Columbia University Press, 1944).
2. Richard Rorty, *Contingency, Irony, and Solidarity* (New York: Cambridge University Press, 1989).
3. John Dewey, *Experience and Nature*, 2d ed., rev. (New York: Dover Publications, 1958), p. 43.
4. Owen Flanagan, "Ethics Naturalized: Ethics as Human Ecology," unpublished manuscript, 1994, p. 7.
5. I owe this point to Flanagan. Ibid., p. 11.
6. Partridge, *Consent and Consensus*, p. 10. The account that follows relies on this source, as well as Elizabeth Flower and Murray G. Murphey, *A History of Philosophy in America* (New York: G. P. Putnam's Sons, 1977).
7. James Q. Wilson, *The Moral Sense* (New York: Free Press, 1993). Sometimes the moral philosophies of Hume, Hutcheson, and Adam Smith, are considered forms of "ideal observer" theory in ethics. The hypothetical ideal observer is absolutely im-

partial and therefore theoretically sets the standard of right and wrong. V. M. Hope, however, argues that they should be viewed as a collectivity of persons with a shared sense of what is fair. See his *Virtue by Consensus*, Oxford: Clarendon, 1989).

8. Wilson, *Moral Sense*, chap. 2.

9. Ibid., chap. 3.

10. Ibid., pp. 40–41.

11. Ibid., p. 11.

12. Paul Churchland, *A Neurocomputational Perspective: The Nature of Mind and the Structure of Science* (Cambridge: MIT Press, 1989), pp. 299–300.

13. My account of states of affairs follows generally from Dewey's discussion of the traits of experience in *Experience and Nature*, chap. 3.

14. For his discussion of the idea of the problematic situation, see John Dewey, *Human Nature and Conduct* (New York: Modern Library, 1930), p. 181 and passim.

15. For a discussion of the idea of social intelligence, see John Dewey, *Liberalism and Social Action* (New York: Capricorn Books, 1963), pp. 67–69.

16. On warranted assertability, see generally John Dewey *Logic: The Theory of Inquiry* (New York: Holt, Rinehart and Winston, 1938).

17. Partridge, *Consent and Consensus*, p. 79.

18. See Charles Bosk, *Forgive and Remember: Managing Medical Failure* (Chicago: University of Chicago Press, 1979).

19. See Robert Zussman, *Intensive Care: Medical Ethics and the Medical Profession* (Chicago: University of Chicago Press, 1992).

20. See Charles Bosk, *All God's Mistakes: Genetic Counseling in a Pediatric Hospital* (Chicago: University of Chicago Press, 1992).

21. Bosk, *Forgive and Remember*, p. 137.

22. Ibid., p. 137 and passim.

23. Ibid., p. 143.

24. Zussman, *Intensive Care*, p. 157.

25. Bosk, *All God's Mistakes*, p. 41.

26. Ibid., p. 42.

8

Small Groups and Social Practices

Philosophical models of group consensus

In speaking of the recent shift in moral philosophy away from a preoccupation with the relation between "a rational, knowing subject and a rationally knowable, objective morality," Bruce Jennings expresses my central concern in this chapter and in the previous one:

[T]he aim is to understand morality as a socially embedded practice, where the crucial questions have to do with the ways in which the meanings and legitimacy of moral notions are established, reinterpreted, and reproduced or transformed over time. What are moral agents doing when they make arguments and counterarguments about what morality requires? This question is now more important than questions about what truth moral knowers can know, and with what degree of certainty. Highlighting moral speech-agency and practice brings consensus and kindred concepts to the fore, as consensus is something moral agents construct, it is not something they contemplatively discover.[1]

The strategy that Jennings describes was applied in the last chapter. In this chapter I formalize this approach to the study of consensus processes as social constructions, focusing on small groups as convenient models of this activity and appealing to discourse theory and "microsociology," the study of small groups. The last part of the chapter addresses some techniques of active intervention in group processes which could be instructive for bioethicists, especially those working in ethics committees and as clinical consultants.

At this juncture it may be helpful to restate my reasons for focusing on the study of actual social practices. Chapter 4 reviewed the rationale for the authority of consensus in a pluralistic society according to the framework of our society's liberal political philosophy. In such a society not all groups will agree with all values, but a stable and predictable overlapping consensus may nevertheless be sustained so long as there is general confidence that common values are respected in the processes of extending moral consensus. Ethics panels (and perhaps some other bioethical institutions such as ethics consultants) often come onto the scene precisely because there is as yet no clear consensus. In those instances we are thrown back upon the integrity of actual consensus processes, where integrity means that those liberal principles that *do* apply are at least honored; in this way perhaps the overlapping consensus can be sustained in the face of new cases and problems. To see how this might be accomplished, we need to know more about actual consensus processes. Thus I have urged that the political rationale for the authority of moral consensus requires supplementation by the study of consensus-oriented practices, a study that contrasts with the rather abstract framework of liberal political philosophy. As a philosophy of bioethics, bioethical naturalism calls attention to these practices as examples of the ways in which moral values emerge from human experience.

The political rationale is concerned with the arrangements of whole societies, but in order to study deliberative consensus processes we need to focus on small groups. The previous chapter offered several examples of how a sociological perspective illuminates certain features of actual small groups. In the abstract, not all of what we have seen is admirable; certainly not all the elements of small group interaction can be credited with contributing to an idea of deliberative democracy or even social intelligence. The more the inadequacies of small groups as sites of moral consensus processes can be identified, the greater are the opportunities to enhance the prospects for deliberative democracy under the rubric of liberal pluralism. Let us now step back to a more philosophical discussion of models of small group consensus processes.

Before I proceed, it will be useful to have a serviceable understanding of the idea of a small group. My rough formulation is that a group may be considered small so long as each member is able to survey all of the other individual group members. This "surveyability" criterion is as precise as the subject permits. Along these admittedly rough lines, Georg Simmel claimed that for hundreds of years this was an important condition for the system of European aristocracy and self-consciousness of its members as part of a small group.[2]

Simmel was a late nineteenth-century sociologist and philosopher who pioneered in small group theory; we will return to his seminal views shortly. Although sociology and philosophy have since divided, philosophers have recently taken up the subject. Among philosophical models of small group consensus, Keith Lehrer's arguments concerning "consensual rationality" are among the most highly developed. He asks us to consider the iterated averaging of the personal probabilities of the group members, or their individual estimates of the likelihood that a certain proposition is true, and then weigh this result in terms of the various degrees of respect the group members have for one another. In the limit case this will lead to a "consensual probability." According to Lehrer, "under expected conditions personal probabilities will coincide with consensual probabilities and consensual probabilities will coincide with the truth."[3] At least two assumptions are implicit in this formulation: first, that people tend to identify correctly who is an expert and who is not, and second, that those who are expert tend to be able to identify true propositions.

Lehrer's formulation does appear to capture the greater part of our intuitions about consensus. It has the virtue of entertaining both the likelihood of a proposition's being true and the effect of knowledgeable members' opinions on the rest of the group. Yet Lehrer's is not a model of an open or information-seeking group, as Peter Caws has pointed out, and indeed it was originally intended to apply to a consensual ranking of alternatives.[4] But a set of discrete alternatives cannot always be provided or even arrived at by a group. Lehrer's concept of consensus is a static one. It has a good deal in common with the Delphi technique, developed by the Rand Corporation much earlier than either the Lehrer or, as we shall see shortly, the Habermas model. Usually collected anonymously and through correspondence, questionnaire results are distributed to participants in successive rounds, encouraging gradual convergence.

Jane Braaten has contrasted Jürgen Habermas's far more dynamic model of consensual rationality with that of Lehrer, which does not attend to interaction within the group.[5] Habermas's characterization of a discursive process of consensual rationality is worth quoting at length.

Discourse can be understood as that form of communication that is removed from contexts of experience and action and whose structure assures us that the bracketed validity claims of assertions, recommendations, or warnings are the exclusive object of discussion; that participants, themes and contributions are not restricted except with reference to the goal of testing the validity claims in question; that no force except that of the better argument is exercised; and that, as a result, all motives except that of the cooperative search for truth are excluded. If under these conditions a consensus about the recommendations to accept a norm arises argumentatively, that is, on the basis of hypothetically proposed, alternative justifications, then this consensus expresses a "rational will." Since all those affected have, in principle, at least the chance to participate in the practical deliberation, the "rationality" of the discursively formed will consists in the fact that the reciprocal behavioral expectations raised to normative status afford validity to a *common* interest ascertained *without deception*. The interest is common because the constraint-free consensus permits only what *all* can want.[6]

Peter Caws calls this passage "an admirable description of what ought to go on in a committee whose recommendations are to carry the force of a consensus."[7] Yet even this account, though richer than Lehrer's, with its emphasis on discursive interaction, can be expanded. Barry Loewer and Robert Laddaga note that "investigators who agree on a program of research may come to agreement concerning hypotheses by carrying out that research." Thus, consensus may be achieved "by experimentation" as well as "argumentation."[8]

All this adds up to a fairly rich philosophical model of group consensus, but it does not, as Caws notes in his survey of these matters, amount to an answer to the strictly epistemological question whether a consensus so accomplished is "right." Many, if not most, of the deliberations of groups such as committees are based in part not on investigations directly undertaken by the members together but rather on the confidence that members have in the "expert" judgment of other members, who may themselves be required to evaluate the judgments of persons not on that team or committee or even in that institution, such as propositions generally accepted by the community of medical scientists. This is "fiduciary" knowledge, that is, knowledge of the trustworthiness of one's sources of information. Without fiduciary knowledge, and without a high degree of confidence in that knowledge, one might as well toss a coin. But fiduciary knowledge is tied directly to the quality of interpersonal relationships, in the sense that it has to do with assessing the reliability of others as makers of certain judgments.[9]

In the group setting a special burden is thus placed on the relations among the members. Especially when life-and-death matters are involved, Caws writes,

[h]aving fiduciary knowledge in the required sense involves precisely "knowing the reasons for which a person deserves respect as a theorist or scholar." This means that interpersonal relations in [ethics] committees must come in for scrutiny in a new and perhaps unwelcome way.[10]

In a similar vein, Allan Gibbard writes of "claims to authority in judgment," which he locates in what he calls "conversational demands."[11] Conversation involves accepting what the other person says, and though these pressures can be and often are resisted, to the extent that they are not, they invoke norms. By way of the explicit or implicit acceptance of these norms, the participants tend toward convergence of viewpoints. Thus, the scrutiny of the ways in which small groups come to collective opinion is an important part of the study of consensus.

Group process and group product

As we proceed, it should be remembered that the subject of small group relations is for present purposes subordinate to the problem of ensuring that the outcome of group deliberation is of a high quality. One means of assessing the quality of the intellectual products of group processes is in terms of the extent to which they approximate some independent "right answer," assuming for the moment that realism is tenable under some theory. But normally the right answer is not known, and that is why the group has met in the first place; thus, a test of group process is not usually available. In this book I have advocated an alternative strategy for examining the process of the group itself. In practice this approach would be represented by questions such as: Have all relevant facts been gathered? Have all important arguments and points of view been aired? Has the discussion presented equitable opportunities for all group members to participate? And so forth. This approach emphasizes the deliberative process rather than its product, and the advantage is that, especially with regard to ethical problems, one is usually in a better position to evaluate the group process than the group product in and of itself because there is a lack of confidence in any particular independent answer to the question that the product of group deliberation is meant to address. Moreover, as I argued at length earlier, in a liberal and diverse society the authority of the consensus that is achieved by devices such as ethics panels (thus sustaining the overlapping consensus in the face of new problems) turns on the extent to which the society's settled values have been honored in those processes.

So it seems that, in any assessment of the outcome of an ethics panel's work, it is important to look to its deliberative processes. But why should it be assumed that a superior group process will tend to yield a superior product? We are intuitively inclined to believe that a result reached by an intensive, informed, and open group discussion of a difficult ethical problem will be superior to a result reached by, say, the flip of a coin. None of us is prepared to agree in advance to a coin toss in answer to the question whether physician-assisted suicide should be legalized, for example. It is hard to say exactly why we resist such a strategy, but at least two sorts of explanations can be identified. The first is that our ancient intellectual heritage tells us the universe is amenable to human understanding, and that discourse is of the same tissue as reality and can help "unconceal" it, as phenomenologists put it. Arguably the human preference for discourse rather than chance in managing moral questions is an evolutionary product, tied to eons of experience in evaluating problematic situations, a process that has been found to be superior to chance, on the whole.[12] A second sort of explanation appeals to the indirect value for a community of putting some of its members into the position of deliberating about some matters that are of concern to all. In Jennings's words, the process

affirms something important about who we are as a community and about our continuing faith in the broad distribution of common sense and the capacity, *under the right circumstances*, for responsible moral deliberation and judgment. . . . Consensus in the strongest sense of the term happens only when it is seen as a common good to be created, and thus the creation of consensus becomes a special civic intention shared by the participants in the moral dialogue.[13]

What is clear is that, when we are insecure about the conclusion reached by our group, we often reflect on the process; note, for example, Jennings's stipulation of a faith in common sense, which I would modify as a common *moral* sense. Thus, again, I have insisted that consensus should be regarded as a deliberative process rather than simply the product of deliberation. Even in the case of ethics panels, we are at least as likely to reconstruct the process as a way of checking our work as we are to consult the writings of the great moral philosophers. This being the case, it is important for bioethics to be informed by theories and disciplines that can shed light on these matters.

Applied social science and small group decision making

A common criticism of small group deliberation is that it can too easily be infected by social pathologies, leading to a distorted "groupthink."[14] Though it is often well founded, one should not infer from this criticism that small groups can never produce high-quality assessments of problematic situations. There is an important confusion behind this error, namely, that the interpersonal influences in a small group almost invariably create obstacles to thinking clearly together. This bias against small group deliberation is closely related to the skepticism about consensus processes that is part of the Western intellectual tradition. But from the mere fact that each small group has a specific interpersonal structure one cannot infer faulty deliberative processes. Furthermore, the study of small groups enables one to explain why some are functional and some are dysfunctional. Thus, by learning about the structure of a particular group one may be able to design interventions that can improve the quality of the group's work. The ethics panel need be no exception.

Most people who are experienced in positions of leadership or authority have an intuitive "feel" for the way interpersonal relations affect the performance of a group. Teachers in elementary schools often change seating arrangements as their pupils become unruly in certain positions. Managers sometimes change a team's work assignments to stimulate renewed creativity. Committee chairs have their own options if the group's work appears to be faltering for some reason, for example, encouraging greater participation by certain members, carefully selecting particular members for subcommittee assignments, or even introducing new members or, at the extreme, dismissing current members if no alternative presents itself. In all these instances there is an understanding that the internal structure of the group is directly related to the way it does its job.

Work on the theoretical aspects of small group relations has not been a vigorous pursuit of social scientists in recent years, although it was central to the emergence of social psychology and sociology from the late nineteenth to the mid-twentieth centuries. The central insights of these studies—that each small group has its own structure and patterns of interaction—are now widely held assumptions. What seems to have led to the lessening of interest in small group studies in positivist social science is the fact that the conclusions one could draw from them either occupy too high a level of generality about social relations or apply in limited terms to particular groups. Hence, decision-theoretic approaches, typified by the "prisoner's dilemma" paradigm, gained more popularity among social psychologists because they seemed more amenable to statistical generalization. Since my goal is nothing like an axiomatized theory of social psychology, these limitations are of no concern in this book. Instead, the insights to be gained from small group theory and from management theory are informative for a philosophical account of moral consensus grounded in social life. And the analytic techniques that were developed by the study of small groups can be useful for those who are professionally involved in the dynamic consensus processes of groups such as ethics committees and ethics commissions.

Although I alluded to legal processes in chapter 4, I have not taken the jury as a paradigm of small group decision making. Certainly when their processes are not subject to the distortions that infect any small group with a mission, when they are not behaving merely like "twelve angry men (and women)," juries may indeed be exemplars of social intelligence. Juries, however, are also integral parts of a legal system that establishes standards for their deliberations which may have as much to do with needs that are unique to that particular system as with the conditions for consensus processes, such as criteria for a valid conclusion that differ from one jurisdiction to the next. In order not to presuppose elements of consensus that may flow from a specific formalized set of social arrangements with particular needs for the legitimization of its decision, I have avoided focusing on the jury system, but prefer to view small groups in a more generic way.

Georg Simmel's small group theory

Although there has been more recent sociological work of a quantitative nature on small groups, the ideas of the German thinker Georg Simmel (1858–1918) show that even in the older sociology there are resources available for the study of consensus processes in ethics panels. Simmel's most famous work was probably *The Philosophy of Money* (1900), but he is not well known outside of sociology. Simmel's observations about reciprocal relations between individuals in small groups are enormously insightful. In this context I will give only a few examples.[15]

Axiomatic in Simmel's social theory is the proposition that the size of a group has a direct bearing on its qualities, for certain types of interaction will emerge only as the group attains a certain size, and the ways in which the group maintains itself will necessarily change as it grows. Thus, small political parties tend to be more radical than larger ones, since the latter must accommodate a greater range of views and temperaments in order to maintain its cohesion as a group. A corollary is that it is difficult for a radical party to sustain its radicalism as it grows. Not only does this observation have interesting implications for consensus theory, but also it epitomizes Simmel's central insight that the size of a group (its quantity) bears a causal relation to its character (its quality). Another implication is that the laws, offices, and symbols that give cohesion to large groups are in effect surrogates for the direct personal relations possible in small groups.

Simmel points out that the role played by prominent individuals changes as the size of the group changes. In general, a millionaire has less influence in a city of one million than in a city of fifty thousand. In a passage with interesting implications for consensus theory, he offers another example:

If, in a parliamentary party of twenty, there are four who criticize the political program or want to secede, their significance in terms of party tendencies and procedures is different from what it would be if the party were fifty strong and had ten rebels within it: although the numerical ratio has not changed, the importance of the ten in the larger party will in general be greater.[16]

In the latter case the ten-member minority would be large enough to strengthen one another, while this is less likely to occur in the four-member minority, and less likely still for smaller minorities within the same overall ratio. For the same reason one might further hypothesize that the smaller group is more likely to view itself as having reached a consensus with a four-member minority than the larger group with its ten-member minority. Of course, if the absolute numbers are the same but the ratios different, one would reach a different conclusion: two dissidents out of ten are more likely to block consensus than two out of one hundred.

In other comments bearing on the importance of group size for individual behavior, Simmel observes that social gatherings of two or three persons require far less mutual adaptation than social gatherings of thirty:

Common traits, which make up the content of sociability among these few individuals, may include such comprehensive or refined aspects of their personalities that the gathering attains a character of spiritual refinement, of highly differentiated and developed psychic energies. But the more persons come together, the less is it probable that they converge in the more valuable and intimate sides of their natures, and the lower, therefore, lies the point that is common to their impulses and interests.[17]

Here Simmel alludes to the familiar experience that the larger the gathering, the more diluted the shared characteristics of group members. Thus, external trappings become more important for the creation of cohesion, such as food, drink, and costumes. From these observations about social gatherings we can infer that those responsible for organizing meetings of bureaucratic entities such as committees need to consider how relative losses of cohesion owing to group size can be accommodated by external arrangements. Unlike social gatherings, meetings of institutional colleagues are already conditioned by symbolic factors such as the fact of collegiality itself, as well as a degree of common interest in the well-being of the institution. Again, however, sheer group size, as well as the different institutional roles of group members, tends to lessen cohesion.

Simmel also observed qualitative differences between the smallest unit of social life, the dyad, and larger units, beginning with the triad. In the case of the dyad, the loss of one member is the destruction of the group. Furthermore, dyads possess a directness of social relation that can be true of no larger unit. A member of the triad or any larger group can observe relationships between other members, but not in the dyad. The directness of dyadic relations also makes it more likely that, in general, secrets will be kept. The triad introduces the fact of indirect relationships, as two can interact through the third, and the third can mediate relations between the other two. This mediating function can make for very strong units, as there is always a third to render assistance to the others' relationship. Although it is true, as folk wisdom has it, that the triad also includes the possibility of viewing the third as an intruder ("three's a crowd"), it is also important to note that the triad is the smallest group that includes this mediating function: "[I]t is clear that from an over-all viewpoint, the existence of the impartial third element serves the perpetuation of the group."[18] Thus, in principle, a triad located within a larger group can be a very powerful unit.

J. L. Moreno's sociometry

Unlike Simmel, who was interested in philosophical observations about the generic qualities of reciprocal relations, the science of sociometry developed by the Viennese-born psychiatrist J. L. Moreno (1889–1974) was designed to analyze the interpersonal structure of particular small groups. Like most other social scientists educated in his time, Moreno must have been influenced by Simmel, and he uses a number of the latter's concepts, such as the dyad and the triad. Sociometry analyzes the structure of small groups according to patterns of interpersonal choice and rejection. These structures can be exhibited on a "sociogram," a sort of map of relations within the group. In the context of the study of consensus processes, sociometry is especially useful in its ability to exhibit group cohesiveness.[19]

According to sociometric theory, an earmark of cohesion in a small group is the presence of linked triads (a group of three in which each chooses the other two) known as "chains." In general, as there are more unlinked triads, more dyads (a couple in which each chooses the other), or more nonchosen individuals ("isolates"), there is less cohesion. The mere presence of a "star," or frequently chosen group member, is in itself no evidence of cohesion or even of power. For example, a star might be chosen by every group member though none of the other group members chooses one another (a fairly common phenomenon among certain groups, such as mental patients who choose only the therapist), so this would not be considered a highly cohesive group. Or a star may be in a mutual dyad with one other member who is otherwise an isolate. Camouflaged by the star, this "Rasputin" can become the true power center of the group.

Some insights available through sociometric analysis can be exemplified in sociograms of actual classes of schoolchildren from kindergarten to eighth grade. At first glance sociograms of kindergarten classes and eighth grade classes seem more similar than they do after further study. For example, there are many links between boys and girls in the kindergarten sociogram; these become fewer and fewer throughout the elementary grades and then finally increase again by eighth grade. Initially it seems that the two subgroups have come full circle. But on closer inspection one appreciates that in the kindergarten group there are few *mutual* choices between the boys and girls, and hardly any triads. The links are fragile. As one moves through the next several years, the degree of complexity of organization, betokened by the appearance of dyads and triads, gradually increases within the subgroup of boys and the subgroup of girls, even as each group withdraws into itself. The appearance of a few "ambassadors" between the boys and girls is accompanied by more stable relations between the sexes. Finally, there are systematic connections both within and between the two subgroups, as chaining becomes evident.

Immature personalities are incapable of sustaining the highly organized systems of interpersonal relationships needed for social stability. Just as schoolchildren dash physically from one playmate to the next in the schoolyard, so they do in a sociometric sense as well. A young child's "best friend" is subject to frequent change. These dynamics can be neatly captured in a temporal series of sociograms. They are also useful reminders that the group structure itself undergoes an evolution as each novel phenomenon faced by the group alters its response to the next one.

A sociogram can also be used in predicting the results of social processes and, if desired, as a guide for active intervention in the reconstruction of a group. Short of that, a sociometric study can identify potential trouble spots in a group that may be amenable to procedural safeguards. To illustrate the usefulness of sociometric investigation with regard to ethics committees, I have created a sociogram of a hypothetical ethics committee in which each member has been asked to choose or reject up to three other members according to the criterion "With whom would you like to discuss a difficult case?" (see Figure 1).

Note first the powerful triadic structures linking four of the nine committee members. These subsystems are even more formidable when one considers that the four most frequently chosen committee members are also members of this chain: A (nine choices), E (five choices), and B and F (four choices). As the universally chosen person on this criterion, the chairperson A undoubtedly exerts considerable influence. But note that the philosopher, E, the second most frequently chosen member, may not be as effective within the group as that rank would suggest, for he actively rejects C, the surgeon. By contrast, although B, the psychiatrist, received fewer choices, the fact that he does not actively reject anyone and that he has access to the other four as well as to D (via a mutual dyad) suggests a relatively more important role for him than for E.

As a potential subgroup the women in this hypothetical ethics committee are highly disorganized, in spite of the fact that the popular chairperson is a woman. While all the women choose A, none are reciprocated. J, the social worker, cannot even muster three choices and receives only one, as well as one rejection. The administrator, I, selects A, F, and H but is either not reciprocated or is actively

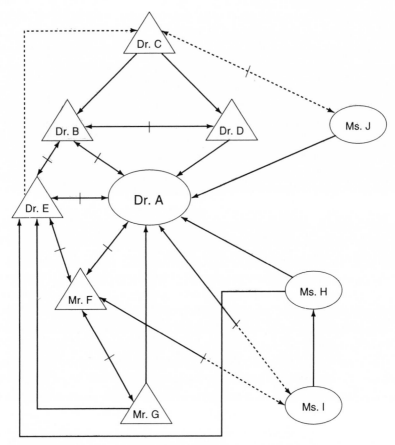

Key:
A: Chairperson, pediatrician, age 44
B: Psychiatrist, 61
C: Surgeon, 46
D: Radiologist, 43
E: Philosopher, 53
F: Lawyer, 35
G: Priest, 48
H: Chief of nursing, 56
I: Administrator, 31
J: Social worker, 48

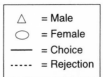

△	= Male
◯	= Female
——	= Choice
-----	= Rejection

Criterion: Discuss a difficult case

OXFORD UNIVERSITY PRESS/MORENO   FIGURE   1   100% BLACK   SIZE   27   X   40

rejected. H is in a very weak position by virtue of being chosen only by J and the isolated I. Yet the surgeon, C, is the most isolated member: he receives no choices, and two members actively reject him.

Not only are sociograms informative about the relations among the members, but they also provide a basis for speculating about the relations among the larger institutional groups of which they are members. In this committee the physician members are relatively integrated, reflecting perhaps the high degree of group consciousness among physicians, while those who come from smaller and less group-conscious constituencies seem to have to reach out to create alliances. Of course, certain social roles have more "natural" mutual sympathies than others, such as chaplains and social workers, and it is therefore a reasonable guess that individuals from these groups will tend to identify with one another on a multidisciplinary panel. All this is not to deny the importance of individual personalities in creating exceptions to these generalizations, but neither should the force of social roles be ignored.

The sociogram can be useful in managing the committee's affairs. For example, the popularity of the chairperson should be monitored so that her formulations do not shape the discussion without some critical assessment. The exclusion of a substantial minority from the tightly organized power structure should be addressed, perhaps by encouraging them to articulate their views early on in deliberating about a particular issue. If subcommittees are ever in order, it will be easy to select from the triads for sheer efficiency. Finally, the sociogram will be most useful if the members of the committee are prepared to overcome their potential embarrassment and resentment at having their relationships so graphically illustrated, for then they will be aware of the interpersonal realities that could inappropriately affect their group processes.

Sociometry is not limited to the analysis of relations within the small group; in principle a sociogram could be constructed that included any finite number of individuals according to some relevant criterion. Indeed, modern computer technology renders this a far more easily realizable possibility than it was in the early days of sociometry, when sociograms mapping the relations among a few hundred individuals had to be constructed laboriously by hand. It is far more practical, however, to design sociograms with human groups rather than human individuals as the relational elements. For example, let us suppose that we are interested in the relationship of our ethics committee to the various other groups within the institution: the medical staff, the nursing staff, the social workers, the chaplains, the administrators, the legal staff, the patient representatives, the risk managers, the board of trustees, and of course the patients. Formally the question could be: "Which groups choose to consult the ethics committee?" Let us suppose that the functional criterion is whether these groups (according to the acts of its individual members who are not on the committee) have interacted with the committee in some way, such as referring a matter for consideration or requesting an "in-service" presentation. There could be a spectrum of choice from relatively frequent (e.g., more than four times a year) to never. Naturally a statistician's help would be needed in weighting the measures of individual groups. For example, some individuals in any group may be heavy users, and a single request for assistance may come from more than one source. These are relatively familiar confounding variables for which statistical techniques have been devised. In this manner the sociometry of an institution in terms of the groups that constitute it can be elucidated.

Management theory and facilitated processes

Although I will not dwell on management theory, the improvement of a group's product by no means requires focusing directly on its internal structure. Often one can work the other way around: exercises designed to improve the group's work product may simultaneously stimulate the group to find new ways to function together. Thus, work in applied social science has also contributed specific procedural protocols to improve the results of small group decision making. For example, there is social psychological evidence that the quality of consensus decision making can be enhanced if the process is rational and systematic. This is said to be necessary because groups are capable of unanimously agreeing on an incorrect solution to a problem, mainly because they have failed to consider all feasible alternatives.[20]

What is known as a "vigilant" group decision-making strategy includes several steps: (1) obtain as much information as possible about the alternatives; (2) thoroughly discuss the value of each alternative; (3) after evaluating the alternatives, rank them according to the most and least desirable; (4) if there is an unranked middle range of alternatives, discuss and rank them; and (5) systematically reconsider the rank assigned to each alternative, without hesitating to change a rank if that is warranted.[21] It is clear that this sort of systematic procedure would have to be adapted to the unique role of the ethics committee. For instance, one alternative the committee will want to consider and rank from time to time is that of giving no advice at all.

Numerous strategies for the improvement of small group functioning through management theory have been developed and utilized by industrial psychologists. Considering the prevalence of ethics panels in bioethics and the immediate effects that distorted interpersonal relations can have on these deliberations, bioethicists have a professional responsibility to learn more about this field. Indeed, in comparison to the relative remoteness of "deep" ethical theory in most actual ethics deliberations, knowledge about small group theory and technique seems at least as important as education in moral philosophy for bioethical deliberation in small groups.

Bioethics can also benefit from knowledge about techniques for intervention in particular cases. The activities of ethics committee members and ethics consultants could fruitfully be considered from the vantage point of alternative dispute resolution (ADR). Although ADR is also a fairly new field, both its conception and its training standards are far better developed than those of ethics interventions. Through a neutral third person ADR applies various methods to mediate and facilitate settlements among interested parties, including a several-stage mediation process and communication techniques. There are quite a few models of facilitated processes: shuttle facilitation, in which the mediator meets separately with the parties as a liaison; mediation, in which several individuals representing the contending viewpoints are brought together; and large group facilitation, when larger numbers of parties with relevant positions are involved.[22]

Several writers in bioethics have suggested that, with important qualifications, facilitated processes could have a role in ethics committee work. The qualifications stem from the different assumptions of ADR and clinical ethics. For example, bioethics tends to render its issues in the language of "dilemma" rather than "dispute."[23] This is consistent with the fact that, as I have noted, consensus is a more usual bioethical framework than compromise. Following from the conflict assumption, facilitation is concerned with correcting for power imbalances among the participants; ethics committees rarely make this a prime consideration. Moreover, some forms of facilitation permit and even encourage the parties to establish their own ground rules at the outset. This would be unrealistic in highly regulated settings such as hospitals, potentially removing the parties from objective constraints such as laws that represent a broad societal consensus.[24]

Nevertheless, following the work of Mary Beth West and Joan McIver Gibson, one can easily see how facilitated processes could be redesigned to fit with the assumptions and goals of ethics committees. Members could be liaisons, as in shuttle facilitation, or small or large group mediators. In all cases the committee would seem well advised to adopt the staged approach that facilitation has developed. The first stage is intake, in which the issue is diagnosed and the process of its resolution is identified. The case consultation stage involves both matters of form, such as where the consultation is to be held, and process, or how the consultation can meet its goals. These will depend on whether the issue is to be resolved or only explored, and whether the committee sees an educational role for itself. The third and last stage is follow-up, or "debriefing" the parties after the episode has passed and offering further assistance.

There are rich possibilities for interaction between the fields of dispute resolution and bioethics. Up to now they have been somewhat divided not only by assumptions and goals but also by the professions and temperaments of the specialists. A growing number of lawyers and social workers are becoming interested in mediation, and they are likely to be the primary bridges between the fields. Furthermore, if a consensus-oriented approach to understanding the social institution of bioethics takes hold, with the result that bioethics is seen partly as a social reform movement (as I will argue in the next and final chapter), there will be greater interest in the lessons of facilitated processes for bioethics.

Witnessing consensus

In this chapter I have mainly been concerned with describing philosophical models and sociological theories of small group processes, and with mentioning some active interventions that might be undertaken by bioethicists. My aim has been to call attention to a dimension of small group processes that can enlarge our understanding of the institution of modern bioethics. Many bioethical activities, and many interventions by bioethicists in the clinical setting, occur in the context of a small group. The group need not be an ethics panel; it could be a gathering of the family of an incapacitated patient and her health care team. Some of the ideas presented in this chapter apply mainly to the ethics panel, and some to these other kinds of small groups.

The notion of introducing dispute resolution methods into the repertoire of the bioethicist should not detract from an appreciation of more "passive" roles of the bioethicist in the quest for moral consensus, especially in the clinical setting. For example, in his study of genetic counselors Charles Bosk reports that he, an anthropologist, was often placed by the counselors in a position that he described as "witnessing":

In a curious way I came to symbolize for the group the moral community outside the hospital—my presence in highly problematic situations became a sign of approbation from the larger community. At one level this exacerbated my difficulties giving the group negative feedback, but it resolved them at another. I could speak as "segments" of the community and raise any objections in a voice that did not seem to be my own.[25]

Not only is Bosk's experience recognizable to bioethicists, perhaps especially those who, like me, are neither doctors nor lawyers, but also in my experience the bioethicist's presence is often sought by harried physicians to *legitimize* a practical discussion of a tough ethics case. On several occasions I have been asked to sit on committees concerning various issues, not all of them primarily ethical in nature, as though my presence would give a sort of secularized moral blessing to the proceedings.

In an illuminating essay George Agich expresses the significance of witnessing as one of the bioethicist's roles:

The role of witness brings the person doing clinical ethics *into* the practice in an intimate fashion; he participates in rather than simply observes the social definition of reality. In effect, the witness is socialized in the practice in question in such a way that he reflects the process of socialization, its definition of reality and its important values and beliefs back to the participants in the practice, thereby validating the sense of reality of the practice, insofar as the witness is not accepted totally within the practice.[26]

Ironically, so long as the witness is perceived as an outsider or "stranger," she can play this symbolic role, but that is a capacity that is lost if she comes to be perceived simply as another member of the group. For the bioethicist in the clinical setting there is a value in remaining an outsider in the perceptions of clinicians.

Arguably there is value in this status for the bioethicist as well. For although no individual can sustain the pure standpoint of an ideal observer, a degree of detachment seems in order for those cast in the symbolically loaded position of "ethicist." One way to achieve this critical detachment (including a healthy dose of self-criticism) is by entering the situation armed with an observational tool kit. Representative items in that kit that have been described in this chapter include both theories and techniques for analyzing small group dynamics in relation to consensus processes, and also for intervening in those processes.

Keeping bioethics pure

Many who are willing to concede that the perspectives discussed in the last two chapters are intellectually interesting may nevertheless fail to perceive their importance for bioethics. Some may even regard the introduction of techniques for analysis of or active intervention in small group processes as pernicious for a field such as bioethics. After all, bioethics has made an enormous contribution, and gained great credibility, from a posture that emphasized the conceptualization of moral problems, using materials derived mainly from philosophy, theology, and the law. Moreover, the incorporation of ideas and techniques from social theory and applied social science threatens to place still greater demands on the already extraordinary requirements for competence in clinical ethics in particular, which include a degree of comfort with the languages of several disciplines.

The situation might be analogized to the evolution of the physician's role over the last five hundred years which has been so well described by the medical historian Stanley Joel Reiser. Where once the physician carefully distinguished himself from the surgeon, who touched patients, used instruments, and was guided by experience rather than philosophy, physicians gradually came to recognize the value of direct contact with patients, devices such as stethoscopes, and theories based on observation. The physicians' descent from their lofty perch revolutionized medicine even as it created new stresses and strains within the profession and in relations with patients and with society as a whole.[27]

In the next chapter I will argue that the "descent" of bioethics from the seminar room to the hospital conference room and the bedside has already made important changes in what began as a more rarefied intellectual pursuit. The import of self-awareness of the "witness" role so artfully described by Bosk and Agich suggests how involved the bioethicist has become in these settings. Furthermore, I believe that bioethics has never been "pure," in the sense that it has always been strongly associated with certain ideas that implicated it in the reform of medicine as a social institution. If this is correct, then the kinds of questions that naturally arise at this point, such as the extent to which the bioethicist should be an agent of consensus and what the implications of such a posture are for the field, are really only bioethics gone self-conscious.

Notes

1. Jennings, "Possibilities of Consensus," p. 448.
2. *The Sociology of Georg Simmel*, ed. Kurt H. Wolff (New York: Free Press, 1950), p. 90.
3. Keith Lehrer, "Personal and Social Knowledge," *Synthèse* 71, 1 (1987): 87.
4. Peter Caws, "Committees and Consensus: How Many Heads Are Better than One?," *Journal of Medicine and Philosophy* 16, 4 (1991): 379.
5. Jane Braaten, "Rational Consensual Procedure: Argumentation or Weighted Averaging?," *Synthèse* 71, 3 (1987): 347–54.
6. Jürgen Habermas, *Legitimation Crisis* (Boston: Beacon Press, 1975), pp. 107–8.
7. Caws, "Committees and Consensus," p. 380.
8. Barry Loewer and Robert Laddaga, "Destroying the Consensus," *Synthèse* 62, 1 (1985): 93.
9. Caws, "Committees and Consensus," p. 389.
10. Ibid., p. 390.
11. Gibbard, *Wise Choices, Apt Feelings*, p. 172.
12. Jeff Blustein helped me see the importance of making this point, and Ruth Macklin suggested the coin-toss illustration.
13. Jennings, "Possibilities of Consensus," p. 461; emphasis added.
14. Lo, "Behind Closed Doors."
15. From *The Sociology of Georg Simmel*.
16. Ibid., p. 98.
17. Ibid., p. 112.
18. Ibid., p. 152.
19. J. L. Moreno, *Who Shall Survive?* (Beacon, N.Y.: Beacon House Publishers, 1953).
20. R. Y. Hirokawa, "Does Consensus Really Result in Higher Quality Group Decisions?," in *Emergent Issues in Human Decision Making*, ed. G. M. Phillips and J. T. Wood (Carbondale: Southern Illinois University Press, 1984).
21. Ibid., pp. 40–49.
22. Mary Beth West and Joan McIver Gibson, "Facilitating Medical Ethics Case Review: What Ethics Committees Can Learn from Mediation and Facilitation Techniques," *Cambridge Quarterly of Healthcare Ethics* 1, 1 (1992): 63–74.
23. Ibid., p. 68.
24. Diane E. Hoffmann, Mediating Life and Death Decisions," unpublished manuscript, 1993.
25. Bosk, *All God's Mistakes*, p. 13.
26. George Agich, "Clinical Ethics: A Role Theoretic Look," *Social Science and Medicine* 90, 4 (1991): 391.
27. Stanley Joel Reiser, *Medicine and the Reign of Technology* (New York: Cambridge University Press, 1978).

9

Bioethics as Social Reform

Taking consensus seriously

In this book we have seen that the importance of moral consensus in bioethics is transparent if bioethics is viewed as an institution and in terms of actual social practices. I first described the scope of the current bioethical consensus and then outlined some of the conceptual considerations relevant to moral consensus. I then argued that, in a society such as ours, the moral authority of consensus in bioethics must be understood within the framework of the liberal political philosophy to which our society subscribes. The challenges that our society's diversity of values presents to this authority were also conceptualized under that rubric. After giving some examples of systematic and self-conscious processes of moral consensus in bioethics by way of ethics panels, I offered bioethical naturalism as a perspective from which the possibility of moral consensus and the qualities that can give it authority in a liberal and diverse society could be examined. Further investigation of routine ethical decision making in clinical settings and of small group processes showed that the importance of bioethical consensus is not limited to formal ethics panels and that its study involves perspectives available in social psychology and sociology.

What remains is to assess the implications of a consensus-oriented account of bioethics for our understanding of bioethics as an institution. To this end I argue that, once the importance of moral consensus processes in bioethics is acknowledged, bioethics cannot be seen simply as the moral philosophy of medicine and health care. I construct a view of bioethics as a social reform movement, contrasting this understanding with an idea of bioethics as a form of advocacy. There follows an outline of the ways in which a deeper appreciation of the role of consensus in bioethics can help it more effectively accomplish its goals as a social reform movement. We then return to the relation between moral consensus and moral expertise. The complexities of the relationship between these two concepts are embodied in the role of the ethics consultant. I conclude with some thoughts about the contribution a bioethics of consensus makes toward managing moral uncertainty in a secular and pluralistic society.

Bioethics as social reform

As a thought experiment consider an alternative universe in which bioethics is strictly an academic pursuit. In this universe there are no ethics commissions authorized by governments, no ethics committees in hospitals. Although there are laws governing certain aspects of physician-patient relations, they are promulgated by nonacademic lawyers, legislators, consumer groups, and professional societies. Although courts of law hear cases involving what we in our universe think of as ethical issues in health care, judges do not consider views beyond those of precedent or judicial philosophy, or of citizens' groups and physicians' organizations. Professors teach courses in the moral philosophy of medicine, but they are not consulted as experts on matters being legislated or tried. Graduating medical students numbly recite some version of the Hippocratic oath at commencement, but they are not systematically exposed to theories of medical ethics.

This scenario strains the imagination, for it obliges us to think of society, even that beyond the academy and the health care system, as very different from the way it is at the end of the twentieth century. Moreover, it presupposes a bifurcation between the academy and the formation of social policy which is quite alien to current practice, at least in the developed world. So profound has been the effect of modern medicine on nearly every aspect of our lives in the past thirty years that we can barely imagine that deeper reflections on it and reactions to it could be limited to the seminar room. Bioethics, as we have come to understand it, is organically related to the changes contemporary generations have witnessed. In point of fact it could no more be amputated from actual social practices than estate planning could be conducted without reference to tax law.

The psychological difficulties of executing this thought experiment themselves make a certain point: the meanings we are so accustomed to ascribing to the idea of bioethics would be absent in the alternate universe. Bioethics is so deeply enmeshed in the drastic social and scientific changes of recent years that it hardly makes sense to think of one without the other. The depth of this involvement can be described in three ways, each expressible by reference to consensus. First, bioethics may articulate an emerging consensus, as when it endeavors to express just what view of some difficult question the bulk of the public is prepared to accept. But a merely descriptive bioethics would not capture the idea as we have become accustomed to it. Thus, second, bioethics may criticize a prevalent consensus, usually by bringing to light some questionable but hitherto unexamined common practice. It does this by contrasting that practice with a widely accepted moral value with which it is in conflict. But again, as important as this function is, critical bioethics still does not wholly satisfy our understanding of bioethics. So, third, bioethics may recommend a new consensus by reasoning to a relatively novel conclusion. A complete account of bioethics in our universe must include prescriptive bioethics.

I offer this typology not for its own sake but by way of supporting a larger point. Founded on efforts to evaluate philosophically current practices in health care, and in light of the results of those evaluations, the institution of bioethics also recommends specific reforms in those practices or describes new practical options, or at least it often does so. Therefore bioethics is inextricably linked with actual social change, and not only in the sense that it evaluates the moral implications of those changes; it is also an agent of social change, of social reform. Although this need not have been the case, it is in fact a proper part of what we have come to understand as bioethics. Moreover, since bioethics has in practice attached itself to a particular set of themes in social reform, including but not limited to the reform of medical education, it can be called a social reform movement.[1]

Engage now in another thought experiment. In a second alternate universe everything is the same as in ours except that bioethics is not identified with the idea of self-determination, either in research or in therapy. Instead there are deep and persistent rifts within bioethics between those who advocate self-determination and those who advocate paternalism in physician-patient relations. To say the least, this has not been the case in bioethics in our universe, and it is an interesting if somewhat tangential additional question whether anyone who consistently advocated a strident paternalism would be considered by the bioethics community to be one of them. In any case, the present point is that self-determination is an abiding theme of bioethics, and the field would surely be quite different were this not so. Insofar as self-determination is a theme that is, in fact, part of the way bioethics is understood, and insofar as bioethics strives to advance this theme in its critical and prescriptive activities, bioethics is a movement. And it is a movement because it is *thematic* in its activities as an agent of social reform.

Probably there are other themes in bioethics that distinguish it from traditional medical ethics, but self-determination is far and away the most obvious and prominent one. Now, taken to an extreme, social reform movements can become advocacy movements. Thus, the patients' rights movement is also quite evidently characterized by a commitment to self-determination, but in that case to say that self-determination is more than a theme of the movement would be an understatement. Rather, for the patients' rights movement self-determination is an *agenda*.

At some point commitment to a theme is qualitatively transformed into commitment to an agenda, and those who are thus committed fall into a special category of social reformer called an *advocate*. What distinguishes the two is this: whereas social reformers are prepared to engage from time to time in public in a critical analysis of their theme, the role of advocate does not in itself permit criticism of the agenda, at least not in public.

Consider specific organizational examples that support this analysis. The Hastings Center is a research institute in bioethics; the Hemlock Society is an advocacy organization for the rights of the terminally ill. Both are closely identified with concerns about self-determination, but in very different ways. In its publications and presentations the Hastings Center pursues this and other broad themes in bioethics, often recommending ways to implement those themes, as in its *Guidelines for the Termination of Life-Sustaining Treatment*.[2] But it also engages in critical analysis of this and other themes. By contrast the Hemlock Society supports specific legislation such as that on assisted suicide to implement self-determination, as the Hastings Center does not, and works hard to let the general public know about its legal rights in these matters, as well as to challenge the law when it fails to conform to its agenda. The former is satisfied to raise questions about bioethics, nearly always thematized by an underlying concern with self-determination. The latter is committed to advancing a certain view about ethics in health care, and is prepared to serve as a strenuous advocate of that view. Of course, individuals who are associated with one organization or the other might sometimes wear one or another hat, but an advocate would not be a good match for the Hastings Center, and an analyst would not be a good match at the Hemlock Society. One implication of this account, for what it is worth, is that the roles of bioethicist and advocate are not only distinct but incompatible.

It would be useful to have a better understanding of the role of a theme such as self-determination in the social reform movement called bioethics. As in a work of art or a public address, a theme is a kind of glue that holds the disparate elements together. The nature of morality in research, the obligations of doctors to patients, the limits of the state in public health crises, the interests of future human beings whose chromosomal constitution might be subject to genetic manipulation are all familiar problems in the bioethical corpus. Self-determination thematizes them in the sense that it helps make them part of the same subject matter. If it does not do that work for all topics in bioethics, or does not do it to the same extent or in the same way, it as at least an organizing principle. As a social reformer the bioethicist is engaged in a movement that seeks to bring to the attention of professionals and the general public the importance of subjects that are so thematized. But since self-determination is a theme rather than an agenda, the bioethicist also maintains an intellectual distance from the single-minded promotion of self-determination, or of a particular conception of self-determination. If she does not, she has become an advocate.

The ready criticism of my analysis comes from counterexamples. Daniel Callahan, Arthur Caplan, Jay Katz, Ruth Macklin, and Robert Veatch, to name a few, are surely all viewed as bioethicists, and all are identified with strong positions on specific bioethical matters. But the point is not that bioethicists never take strong positions and stick to them. Rather, in presenting a reasoned defense of their views, they are implicitly prepared to entertain other views, and this is mandatory in their role as bioethicists. Were they simply advocates, they would not be so prepared, nor would it be mandatory for them to be. Finally, this analysis is not an attack on advocacy but an attempt to distinguish it from social reform. By and large I am an admirer of the work of patients' rights advocates (though not usually that of the Hemlock Society), and I hope that at least some of what I write and say as a bioethicist is valuable to them in the pursuit of their agendas.

Bioethics, the moral philosophy of medicine, and medical ethics

In this section I want to expand on an experience that is familiar to bioethicists working in so-called applied settings. It has been particularly well expressed by the first philosopher to teach in a medical school, K. Danner Clouser, in the context of a discussion of the role of cases in teaching ethics. Although Clouser's remarks are directed at the difference between the use of cases in the seminar and in the clinical conference, he illustrates a larger point about the contrasting nature of moral deliberation in each situation:

Trying out one's theory on real situations, thick with details, is very different from the philosopher's typical hypothetical case, which, if not simply invented, is so highly abstracted from real circumstances that only enough details remain to defend selectively the particular point the philosopher wants to make thereby. His or her use of cases is much more to *illustrate* theory than to test it. But when *solving* the moral problem is the main point, the relentlessness of the details becomes readily apparent. There is no refuge; there is one quagmire after another; retreating to the theory is not a viable option.[3]

Further interesting results follow from consideration of the role of consensus in bioethics. In particular, through the lens of consensus the social reform elements of bioethics become more obvious, and more obviously important, especially in certain "applied" settings. Just how important are the social reform elements of bioethics? To some extent the first thought experiment in the previous section already answered this question: without these elements bioethics would simply not be the field we understand it to be in the late twentieth century. To make this point a bit clearer, we can contrast bioethics (or biomedical ethics) with the moral philosophy of medicine and with what might be called traditional medical ethics.

The moral philosophy of medicine refers to instruction in ethical issues in medicine and health care which is undertaken as part of a formal course of study. Sometimes this kind of instruction takes place under the rubric of course titles such as "Present Moral Problems" or "Ethical Issues in Health Care" or even "Bioethics"; philosophers use what Clouser calls "typical hypothetical cases" in these courses. As in any field of study in the liberal arts (and bioethics is really a multidisciplinary field rather than a discipline), the primary purpose is to open the minds of students to possibilities they had not considered, to liberate them from their prejudices. Consensus among the students about the issues examined in the course is not a primary goal of the class, and may even be regarded as undesirable by diehard Socratic educators, who stress the importance of reasoned disagreement as a way of stimulating thought.

Now, compare this context to that of a clinical case conference in a teaching hospital in which the topic is some perceived ethical issue in an ongoing case, the sort of situation in which, as Clouser puts it, one often confronts "one quagmire after another." Normally the house officers sit with several attending physicians in a session led by someone recognized by the group as an "ethicist," and often the matter is so pressing that some conclusion must be reached by the end of the session, a conclusion that implies what specific actions will be taken and by whom. Although instruction is a highly desirable feature of clinical ethics conferences, as it is for all the activities in which physicians in graduate training are participants, the primary purpose is to formulate a consensus about what is to be done. Just as pedagogical processes tend to shape the seminar in the moral philosophy of medicine, consensus processes tend to shape the clinical ethics conference. It hardly needs to be said that this is even more the case in ethics committees and commissions. Of course there are sometimes mixed cases, as in a more formal academic presentation (perhaps a grand rounds), in which there is less pressure to decide about the ethical management of a "live" case and more room for the presenter to array alternative points of view without necessarily endorsing any one in particular.

I am not suggesting that the moral philosophy of medicine, represented in formal courses of study in colleges and universities, is not a part of the social institution we call bioethics. Rather, I contend that it is only contingently so, for if our universe were instead the one sketched in the beginning of the previous section, there would be studies in the moral philosophy of medicine without there being an institution that we in our universe have come to call bioethics. Of course, all liberal arts education can be regarded as a kind of social reform, since it is an article of faith in the liberal arts that liberally educated citizens will prefer a different sort of society from that which citizens who are not so educated would be prepared to accept. But this is social reform in a rather indirect and extended sense.

Now, consider the traditional institution of medical ethics. In using this expression I refer to medical ethics as an instrument of social control that characterized the medical profession for centuries. This sense of the term survives in the form of peer review, especially in cases of egregious professional misconduct about which there is no room for serious disagreement: sexual relations with patients is perhaps the most prominent example. Historically, traditional medical ethics was a device that helped constitute the social boundaries of the medical profession, distinguishing those who were in the fraternity from those who were not. Those who were among the initiated were only those persons who had pledged to adopt certain patterns of suitable conduct (or virtue). In practice these patterns of conduct were less *studied* than they were *conveyed* by example (role modeling) from one generation to the next. Although there were of course great thinkers in medical ethics before modern bioethics, such as Percival, Gregory, and Bernard, their works and innovations were received not as inspirations for further discussion so much as further adumbrations of the implicit obligations of the physician. They became part of the medical fraternity's ethical consensus, but they were not received in such a way that they stimulated further reflection. To be sure, it could have been otherwise; but the quasi-militaristic and hierarchical educational traditions of medicine did not permit the give-and-take of the liberal arts environment. Traditional medical ethics, in other words, was intended to give substantive guidance to physicians, not to open their minds to the free play of ideas. Indeed, medical (and legal) education is often called training, a revealing term that distinguishes it from liberal arts traditions, which stress methods of thinking rather than technique.

It seems to me that the modern field of bioethics embraces both ends of this particular spectrum, for it includes the moral philosophy of medicine, in which consensus is not a goal, as well as medical ethics in its traditional sense, in which consensus is crucial. Both ends of the spectrum persist, of course, but there is a tendency to overidentify bioethics with one end or the other. If bioethics is identified as the moral philosophy of medicine, its consensus-oriented elements are left out; if it is identified with medical ethics, critical and reflective elements are ignored. What ties the extremes together and gives bioethics its special character is precisely all of the activities between these two extremes, activities that are a marvelously rich blending of philosophical analysis and criticism and social interventionism.

This account has implications for the social roles of bioethicist, moral philosopher of medicine, and medical ethicist. The moral philosopher of medicine is, in the first instance, a moral philosopher. Skills associated with consensus processes are not expected of the moral philosopher and, given a sufficiently Socratic view of the nature of philosophy in human affairs, are even anathema to the moral philosopher's task. The medical ethicist, as I believe the term should be used, is one who is expert in identifying the prevailing professional norms of medical practice. The medical ethicist could be called on by a peer review body or a court of law to describe the ethical standards that would apply under particular circumstances, as when a physician stands accused of inappropriate conduct with a patient. Now, the bioethicist is one who might well be able to play both of these roles but is especially adept at identifying and explicating controversial issues. In doing so the bioethicist is expected to be able to defend a particular conclusion, as the moral philosopher of medicine might not be expected to do (Socratic educators like to leave their students hanging), and critically analyze their own position as well as prevailing norms, as the medical ethicist might not be expected to do (lawyerly medical ethicists need not be self-critical).

Ethics consultation

During the past two decades, and accelerating recently, a new professional role has been introduced into a number of hospitals. Ethics consultants, working with or without an ethics committee, may be retained by administrators to provide expert services to clinical staff concerning ethically controversial treatment choices. I am not speaking here of ethics consultation services provided by ethics committees, usually in the form of on-call subcommittees. Rather, I consider the salaried clinical ethics consultant a related but distinct phenomenon.

Viewed again from a consensus-oriented conception of bioethics, the ethics consultant's role is especially interesting. In some respects the ethics consultant is both a moral philosopher of medicine and a medical ethicist, as I defined these terms earlier. More central to this role, however, is the fact that the ethics consultant is a novel sort of clinician, bringing ethical analysis and intervention to the bedside. The ethics consultant helps make patient self-determination a theme of clinical decision making and is in that sense a bioethicist. In this respect the ethics consultant is engaged in social reform, particularly in the reform of physician-patient relations, with the locus that of particular cases. The ethics consultant must also retain an analytic posture and critical distance that is also typical of the bioethicist; otherwise, she has an agenda rather than a theme and becomes indistinguishable from the patient advocate down the hall.

It is possible to identify two approaches to ethics consultation. On the first or "soft" model, the ethics consultant is largely a facilitator, bringing together the relevant parties, helping to sort out the facts, clarifying the problem at hand, raising important moral questions, and noting useful distinctions.[4] The emphasis is largely casuistic. On the second or "hard" model, the ethics consultant behaves more like a traditional clinician, undertaking an independent investigation that includes an examination and interview of the patient or perhaps the family, insofar as that is possible, and issuing a recommendation. Although some aspects of the first model may be utilized, they are largely subordinate to a reasoned analysis of the alternatives based on an application of ethical principles.[5]

Although it is tempting to characterize the first model as reflecting a consensus orientation and the second as representing an emphasis on expertise, this conclusion would be superficial. While it is certainly true that a consultant on the first model is more obviously up to building consensus than the second, the first kind of consultant fails if she does not present a case that is sufficiently persuasive to generate a consensus. Conversely, if the second kind of consultant does not convey a sense of expertise in clinical ethics, then she can hardly expect to enjoy the confidence of busy colleagues, suffering patients, and worried families. Both consultation models require a degree of perceived expertise and are consensus development processes, albeit with differing emphases.

The first model of ethics consultation might be regarded as an instance of dynamic consensus processes, while the second model renders a more static form of consensus. But what decisively distinguishes even the soft model of ethics consultation from the ethics committee is the fact that the consultant is the administratively designated authority figure when there is ethical uncertainty, regardless of how adept the consultant may happen to be in lightly wielding her power. No individual on the ethics committee can make this claim—unless the consultant is herself a committee member.

Whether or not a member of the committee, a single salaried consultant or a consultation team could work in conjunction with an ethics committee. This sort of arrangement has been described by Stephen Wear and his colleagues. The consultants found themselves developing rules of thumb amounting to informal policies as they continually gained experience with cases. They were uncomfortable with this situation, partly because they did not feel themselves to be sufficiently representative of the institution to legitimate these emerging policies. Thus, an ethics committee was formed to evaluate, formalize, and disseminate the guidelines that were emerging in the course of the consultants' practice. The hybrid system that resulted provides an interesting study in multiple iterated levels of dynamic consensus building involving the consultants, the committee, and the wider institution.[6]

The emergence of ethics consultation is part of a new branch of bioethics called clinical ethics. John Fletcher and Howard Brody have written that in clinical ethics "inquiry tends to start from the reality of a clinician-patient encounter and ends in a practical case judgment which impacts upon an identifiable patient."[7] Clinical ethics has spawned its own literature and professional organization (the Society for Bioethics Consultation), and much of the emphasis of the previous chapter was on interventions that might be undertaken under the clinical ethics rubric. Still, it is significant that clinical ethics represents a pronounced version of tendencies that were latent in bioethics as a social reform movement; it might be said that clinical ethics is a manifestation of bioethics as social reform in the hospital setting.

Ethics consultation and social reform

The ethics consultant is a de facto agent of social reform in a way that the teacher of ethics is not. For the ethics consultant is in a position to do more than teach, criticize, and analyze. Because she is an ethicist, the ethics consultant is well placed to discern hitherto unrecognized ways in which rival belief systems might be adapted (e.g., the adult child who wants "everything done" for her parent with multiple system failure but will consent to a do-not-resuscitate order to avoid vegetative existence); reasonably modified (the surgeon who agrees to delay a risky corrective procedure for a heart defect for an infant with numerous uncorrectable anomalies in order to assess the child's pulmonary potential); or even defensibly constrained (the practice of obtaining court orders to transfuse children of Jehovah's Witnesses). Because she is a consultant in the health care setting, directly engaged in working out acceptable social arrangements in cases such as these, the ethics consultant assumes a role in the "political" processes that are an essential part of the management of tensions among the values of a diverse society.

Beyond a certain point it is useless to wonder whether the ethics consultant should participate in these processes or not. As soon as the individual identified as the "ethics expert" leaves the seminar room or library for the hospital conference room or nursing station, the transformation from moral philosopher to ethicist has been accomplished; that is, the moral philosopher no longer only trades in theory and hypothesis but participates in institutional decision making about particular cases. In these circumstances the ethics consultant must adopt the sanguine posture that the moral philosopher's intellectual abilities can be brought to bear, but not without some additional skills required of participants in human institutions. Thus, the outstanding question is: What skills besides moral expertise does the ethics consultant require? Although this question invites a study in itself, I will briefly offer some suggestions.

It is often said that the nonphysician ethics consultant must be familiar with the language of health care in order to be effective. But there are at least three other sorts of skills that are required for all ethics consultants to play their inherently political role effectively. Some were mentioned at the end of the preceding chapter. They probably all suggest a level of formal training that few ethics consultants can yet claim, but it would be surprising if those who are generally considered successful did not have sound intuitions in these directions. First, the consultant should be a skilled participant-observer, able to identify informal social structures and arrangements and to assess his or her developing role in them. Second, the consultant should understand the dynamics of small group behavior and possess an ability to recognize the interplay between sociometric structures and decisional outcomes. Third, the consultant should be a competent mediator, familiar with negotiating strategies, and having sound interpersonal skills.[8]

Ethics consultation is the most extreme example of bioethics as social reform, and it is the one that shows just how vacuous is the hackneyed concept of applied ethics. The difference between the moral philosophy of medicine and ethics consultation is not simply that between theory and practice, nor even between abstract and concrete. Rather, the difference can best be captured by focusing on the qualitatively different roles of moral philosopher of medicine and ethics consultant, roles that are embedded in social practices and institutional contexts.

The demands of consensus for bioethics

Earlier in this book I explored the usefulness of social analysis for an understanding of moral consensus processes in health care institutions. Ethics consultants intervene more directly in these processes than others who might be considered part of the institution of bioethics; and although I have not attempted to reach any prescriptive conclusions concerning the very idea of ethics consultation, it is a good bet that this practice will be with us for some time to come and that its popularity will grow. For, like ethics committees, ethics consultants provide an opportunity for the socially acceptable management of potentially explosive institutional issues. It is important to note that, like ethics committees, ethics consultants can also help an institution settle problems without resort to the expensive, highly public, and generally unsatisfactory alternative of a court of law. Unlike ethics committees, however, which are founded on the idea of multidisciplinary cooperation, ethics consultation is based on the idea of ethical expertise. Nevertheless, both models require a background conception of consensus processes. On another occasion a distinct problem with the salaried ethics consultant role must be pursued: that is, to what extent is such an individual subject to the pressures of conformity with the institution's interests rather than representation of the themes of bioethics, especially patient self-determination? It is clear, on the view of ethics consultation I have sketched, that these individuals must be scrupulously aware of the dangers of co-optation. Arguably they should be given some sort of formal protection from this danger, perhaps even a form of tenure so that they can retain moral independence from even well-intentioned employers.

The conclusions I have drawn concerning suitable skills for ethics consultants apply as well to ethics committees, namely, that they should have the ability to analyze and intervene effectively in interpersonal relations. These are not skills that are within the basic repertoire of most physicians, philosophers, or lawyers. Since most ethics consultants come from these disciplinary backgrounds, education in social analysis and intervention seems recommended. By contrast, ethics committees normally include individuals who, by background or experience or both, have these kinds of abilities on which the rest of the committee can call, such as nurses, social workers, chaplains, patient advocates, and some psychiatrists and psychologists. Even in those instances, however, it is worth considering whether the standard sorts of educational programs for ethics committee members should be expanded to include training in interpersonal relations.

If I have even modestly succeeded in this book, I will have convinced bioethicists of the importance of moving consensus into the center of their theoretical considerations. I will also have managed to make a convincing case that sociology and social psychology, as well as philosophical models of social processes, are not subjects that are somehow tangential to bioethics. Owing to the nature of bioethics as a social reform movement, intellectual honesty and conceptual adequacy demand that the topics represented in these disciplines be included in the scope of bioethical theorizing.

The limits of consensus for bioethics

I set as the goal of this book a comprehensive account of moral consensus in bioethics for a liberal, democratic, and pluralistic society. Of the many claims that can be filed against this effort are two that I want to address in particular. First, it will perhaps be said that, by viewing bioethics in terms of consensus processes, I am debasing the essentially critical and philosophical character of bioethics, and that I am therefore contributing to the reduction of the field to what Daniel Callahan has called "regulatory bioethics." By this he refers to efforts to find a middle way between supporters and opponents of some practice, and to establish a procedural consensus that eventuates in the regulation of that practice as an agreeable alternative to banning it or not restricting it at all. Regulatory bioethics is contrasted, in Callahan's language, with "prophetic bioethics," or the critique of modern medicine, its practices, and its values. In much the same way that a religious community may be called to its conscience, prophetic bioethics challenges the goals and purposes of practices that might not otherwise be called to account. Regulatory bioethics, by contrast, focuses more on the means of managing potentially controversial practices, with the national commissions as examples.[9]

In this book I have argued for a broader conception of the role of consensus in bioethics, one that moves beyond the more obvious cases of national ethics commissions to ethics committees and routine clinical decision making. The protean nature of consensus enables it to turn up in all sorts of situations and guises, and not only as part of the more formal governmental panel. Unless we come to terms with the importance of consensus in a field such as bioethics, we will not take seriously Philoctetes' challenge.

The distinction between prophetic and regulatory bioethics cannot be taken at face value. A concern for prophecy without a corresponding concern for managing human affairs contains the seeds for much mischief. Of course, no one would admire management without vision, but what about the reverse? What sort of a prophet leads the flock to the golden pasture and then leaves it to its own devices, without guidance? Although Moses did not enter the Promised Land, he left the Law for others to follow. Put less lyrically, in this book I have often expressed doubt about the legitimacy of distinctions based on means and ends, which recall Platonic contrivances. In any case, the concept of bioethics as a social reform movement surely embraces both prophetic and regulatory aspects.

Apart from the implications and merits of this distinction, it does capture the reasonable concern that an overemphasis on process issues could draw away intellectual energy from the larger questions that have so enlivened both academic and popular discourse about medicine. I would not care to contribute to the depreciation of this activity, but neither do I think that a consensus orientation necessarily has that effect. Rather, the study of consensus in bioethics might just as well have the salutary effect to which Callahan alludes. Indeed, the acknowledgment of the role of consensus in bioethics has the potential to encourage this effect in a powerful manner. For one way to call a community to conscience, and thereby to invite collective reflection, is to make its predilections public, as a democratic assembly may be polled for the sense of the house.

Finally, highlighting consensus processes in bioethics is recommended as a corrective to a largely unself-conscious field. Not only the wider society but also the bioethical community itself could benefit from the self-critical possibilities inherent in the call to examine its consensus processes. Even the prophets of bioethics could stand some "nudging" now and then. Indeed, considering how much criticism bioethics has heaped on the institutions of modern health care, including the failure of organized medicine to police itself adequately, it is startling how little bioethics has evaluated its own performance as a social institution.

A second anticipated criticism of my project is that in depreciating the fact-value distinction, I have implicitly advanced an approach to bioethics without moral foundations. In bioethics there is special reason to be concerned about the loss of moral moorings, for modern bioethics operates against the horizon of the involvement of physicians in the exploitation of concentration camp inmates under Nazi Germany. This and the entire Nazi era are often seen as testimony to the dangers of a moral consensus operating without an independent moral standard. I believe, however, that the sources of Nazi doctrine lie not in the dangers of consensus but rather in a dogmatic, absolutist philosophy that combines bad biology with distorted metaphysics. Thus, the Nazis did not lack an independent "moral standard"; the trouble was that the standard they had was hideous.

In any case, understanding bioethics in terms of liberal political philosophy and bioethical naturalism hardly leaves bioethical discourse without foundations. As an institution within the liberal tradition, bioethics calls attention to the tough and ongoing project of protecting individual rights while sustaining justifiable social structures. In offering the idea of the moral sense as an explanatory model for the possibility of consensus, I have argued that there is a "database" for the deeper understanding of moral consensus. Indeed, I have specifically opposed the notion that moral consensus is merely conventional. As to my rejection of a simplistic fact-value dichotomy, even the most admirable moral standard makes no difference in the world if it is not put into practice. The more separate a morality is from the world of human action and experience, the less related to that world it would seem to be. This view is at the heart of bioethical naturalism.

The dangers of consensus for bioethics

In another vein, Callahan's reference to prophetic traditions has great strategic importance for bioethicists. As an implicit form of criticism of the status quo, prophecy can avoid being held accountable for the failures of specific changes.

When a field moves beyond prophecy to become an agent of specific, widespread innovation, it has effectively become part of the "establishment" and thus acquires accountability. Our social and intellectual history includes numerous instances of this phenomenon. The roles of psychiatry in the care of "lunatics," of economics in fiscal policy, and of sociology in social welfare arrangements all exemplify how professions have identified a societal problem, moved into the breach, and then taken their lumps for perceived failures of reform.

As bioethics becomes increasingly identified as part of the health policy and health care establishments, there is no reason to believe that it will be immune from a similar fate. This process could have begun at least as early as the advent of the President's Commission but, except among a few disgruntled physicians who cast aspersions at meddling "ethicists," it has not. One reason why bioethics has avoided the usual accountability of other "applied" fields may be the fact that, unlike psychiatry, economics, and sociology, the field of bioethics is not isomorphic to a particular discipline. Since bioethicists can be philosophers, lawyers, physicians, theologians, nurses, and others, it is somewhat more difficult for particular failures of reform to be associated with them. And of course, again in reference to Callahan's analysis, much of bioethics continues to be prophetic rather than regulatory, and thus relatively refractory to criticism. Nonetheless, the use of the unlovely term *ethicist* has gone a long way toward establishing the popular impression that those to whom it refers are members of a profession, subjecting them also to the expectation that they are constrained by standards of practice.

Although bioethicists have enjoyed wearing the good guy's "white hat" (allowing again for the increasingly rare exception of hostile doctors), this privileged position cannot last forever. Beginning with the influence of governmental and professional bioethics commissions, continuing with the voluntary establishment of ethics committees, and accelerating with committees mandated by professional self-regulation and state and (perhaps in the future) also federal law, bioethics as a distinct field is sure to impress itself more and more on the public mind, and so, therefore, will its inadequacies and failures. The establishment of a professional association that purports to be an umbrella organization for the field (the American Association of Bioethics), will further crystallize this public presence, for well or ill.

There is finally the danger that a bioethical consensus can "sanctify" a certain position, to use Nicholas Rescher's term, and thereby move it beyond serious reconsideration. This worry has surfaced repeatedly in this book, especially in the context of Jay Katz's critique of ethics commissions. In a sense, my entire purpose has been to reduce this possibility by subjecting bioethical consensus to study from various viewpoints. If I am right that consensus processes are an ineliminable part of the institution of bioethics, then this kind of study should become routine in the field.

The virtues of consensus

The sense in which consensus is a double-edged sword was seen most clearly in the chapter on ethics commissions. On the one hand, it is generally recognized that consensus lubricates social and political life, while on the other, it arguably permits matters to proceed too smoothly, thereby masking important underlying conflicts or distracting attention from concerns that deserve to be aired. In scholarly discussions of consensus, its shortcomings tend to receive more attention than its virtues, even when what critics often desire is the replacement of one consensus with another. My view is not that role of moral consensus in the life of a society requires defense, but that it is unavoidable; indeed, readers may find themselves both more aware and suspicious of moral consensus as a result of the arguments and studies in this book.

Nevertheless, the virtues of consensus are considerable, especially when seen in comparison with more formal ways of managing potential uncertainty or conflict about moral issues, such as the law, and when constrained by a respect for personal autonomy and dissent. Certainly not all moral disagreements should be subjected to adjudication or legal codification. There are many reasons for this. A utilitarian reason could be that a legal standard may not, in fact, succeed in achieving the desired result. After all, the law is a fairly heavy and often clumsy hand. Beyond failing to shape conduct as might be wished, legal requirements frequently inspire self-righteous efforts to undermine them. The attempted prohibition of alcoholic beverages is a classic example of this phenomenon in American social history. Alcoholism was a terrible public health problem by the turn of the century, and continued to be after the end of Prohibition, but the police power of the state seemed a poor instrument for turning the tide. After that experience it became a commonplace that the law should not try to get too far ahead of a social consensus that could make it enforceable. Another reason could be the unseemliness of imposing a legal code on moral conduct. Instead of operating under a rubric of competing rights and negotiated compromise (with all its attendant artificially contained tensions), consensus implies a rubric of common interests.

Not all social arrangements should be legally codified, and not all propositions about ethics reach the confidence level necessary to be axiomatic. Bioethics is full of examples, and at least one official reason for creating ethics commissions and committees has been the dramatic moral ambiguities that arise in dealing with novel biomedical technologies. Occasionally when I have presented to physicians on bioethical issues, I have been told that there should be official "protocols" for ethical decision making, especially in legally hazardous areas such as that of abating life-sustaining treatment. Those who make such requests are driven by legal as well as moral worries, but it is still ironic to hear physicians express their willingness to give up even more of the autonomy that was once so precious to the medical profession. Consensus processes are frequently too informal to provide the level of comfort these physicians seek, but they are far superior to rushing to new regulation in contentious territory.

Finally, the study of consensus in bioethics per se can serve as a corrective to an ethnocentric tendency in the field. The medical sociologists Renee C. Fox and Judith P. Swazey delivered a powerful warning about this some years ago, referring especially to the individualistic orientation of American bioethics. Without rehearsing their entire argument, one can suggest its flavor in a single passage:

> Within its rigorously stripped-down analytic and methodological framework, bioethics is prone to reify its own logic and to formulate absolutist, self-confirming principles and insights. These tendencies are associated with the disinclination of bioethics to critically examine its own moral epistemology; to searchingly identify and evaluate the presuppositions and assumptions on which it rests.[10]

This statement was surely more descriptive when it was written, in the mid-1980s, before the debate between principlists and casuists about method in bioethics, and before much attention had been given to the perspectives of ethnic minorities and of feminism concerning bioethical issues. Still, sustained attention to the nature of consensus in bioethics can play an important role in advancing the "critical bioethics" that has stirred since Fox and Swazey's analysis.

My hope is that this book will stimulate further efforts to understand consensus in bioethics. As I have labored to show, consensus is so much a part of our moral and social lives that no reasonably complete account of ethics can do without it. Certainly no reasonably complete account of a social reform movement such as bioethics can afford to ignore it.

Notes

1. John Fletcher's account of bioethics as a social reform movement is in essential agreement with mine, though he places the emphasis on the relation of bioethics to national political trends rather than consensus building. See John C. Fletcher, "The Bioethics Movement and Hospital Ethics Committees," *Maryland Law Review* 50, 3 (1991): 859–94.
2. Hastings Center, *Guidelines for the Termination of Life-Sustaining Treatment and the Care of the Dying* (Bloomington: Indiana University Press, 1987).
3. K. Danner Clouser, *Hastings Center Report*, Special Supplement, 25, 6 (1993): S11.
4. For an example of the first model, see Terrence F. Ackerman, "Conceptualizing the Role of the Ethics Consultant," In *Ethics Consultation in Health Care*, ed. John C. Fletcher, Norman Quist, and Albert R. Jonsen (Ann Arbor: Health Administration Press, 1989), pp. 37–52.
5. For an example of the second model, see John LaPuma and David L. Schiedermayer, "Ethics Consultation: Skills, Roles, and Training," *Annals of Internal Medicine* 114, 2 (1991): 155–60.
6. Stephen Wear et al., "The Development of an Ethics Consultation Service," *HEC Forum* 2, 2 (1990): 75–87.
7. John C. Fletcher and Howard B. Brody, "Clinical Ethics: A New Branch of Biomedical Ethics," in *Introduction to Clinical Ethics*, ed. John C. Fletcher, Charles B. Hite,

Paul A. Lombardo, and Mary Faith Marshall (Charlottesville: University of Virginia School of Medicine, 1994), p. 360.

8. Jonathan D. Moreno, "Ethics Consultation as Moral Engagement, *Bioethics* 5, 1 (1991): 44–56.

9. Daniel Callahan, personal communication, May 17, 1993. See also Daniel Callahan, "Why America Accepted Bioethics," *Hastings Center Report*, Special Supplement, 23, 6 (1993): S8–S9.

10. Renee C. Fox and Judith P. Swazey, "Medical Morality Is Not Bioethics: Medical Ethics in China and the United States," *Perspectives in Biology and Medicine* 27, 3 (1984): 356.

Index